Supplement 1 zu Band 18,
Juni 2002

Chirurgische Gastroenterologie Interdisziplinär

Herausgeber:
E. Klar, P. Schemmer,
Heidelberg

Transplantation: Steigerung der Organverfügbarkeit

Mit freundlicher Unterstützung
durch ***Aventis Behring*** GmbH

KARGER
Basel · Freiburg · Paris · London · New York ·
New Delhi · Bangkok · Singapore · Tokyo · Sydney

Chirurgische Gastroenterologie Interdisziplinär

Supplement 1 zu Band 18, Juni 2002

Gegründet 1984 als «Chirurgische Gastroenterologie mit interdisziplinären Gesprächen» durch A. Akovbiantz, H. Denk, K.-J. Paquet und C. E. Zöckler.

S. Karger · Medical and Scientific Publishers · Basel · Freiburg · Paris · London · New York · New Delhi · Bangkok · Singapore · Tokyo · Sydney

Die Zeitschrift erscheint vierteljährlich: pro Jahr erscheint 1 Band zu je 4 Heften. Bezugspreis für Jahrgang 18, 2002: Euro 144.– / SFr 202,– einschließlich MwSt., zuzüglich Postgebühren. Der Abonnementpreis ist im Voraus zahlbar. Das Abonnement der Zeitschrift läuft weiter, wenn es nicht spätestens 4 Wochen vor Abschluss eines Bandes abbestellt wird.

Abonnementbestellungen können bei jeder Buchhandlung oder direkt beim Verlag aufgegeben werden:

Deutschland:
S. Karger GmbH
Lörracher Str. 16 a
D-79115 Freiburg
Tel. +49 761 45 20 70
Fax +49 761 4 52 07 14
E-mail Information@Karger.de

Übrige Länder:
S. Karger AG
Allschwilerstr. 10
CH-4009 Basel
Tel. +41 61 3 06 11 11
Fax +41 61 3 06 12 34
E-mail Karger@Karger.ch

Anzeigen: S. Karger
Verlag für Medizin und Naturwissenschaften GmbH,
Lörracher Str. 16 a. D-79115 Freiburg, Tel. +49 761 45 20 70.
Gültig ist die Preisliste Nr. 9 vom 1. Januar 2002.

Verlagsleitung und presserechtlich verantwortlich:
Sibylle Hopf
Redaktionsassistenz: Dr. Hannelore Tenckhoff
Anzeigenleitung: Susanne Meister
Produktionsleitung: Georg Brunner

Herstellung: druckhaus köthen GmbH
Friedrichstraße 11/12, D-06366 Köthen/Anhalt

ISBN 3-8055-7378-2

KARGER

Fax +49 761 452 07 14
E-mail Information@Karger.de
www.karger.com

Home Page der Zeitschrift:
www.karger.com/journals/cga

Bibliographische Dienste:
EMBASE / Excerpta Medica
Reference Update

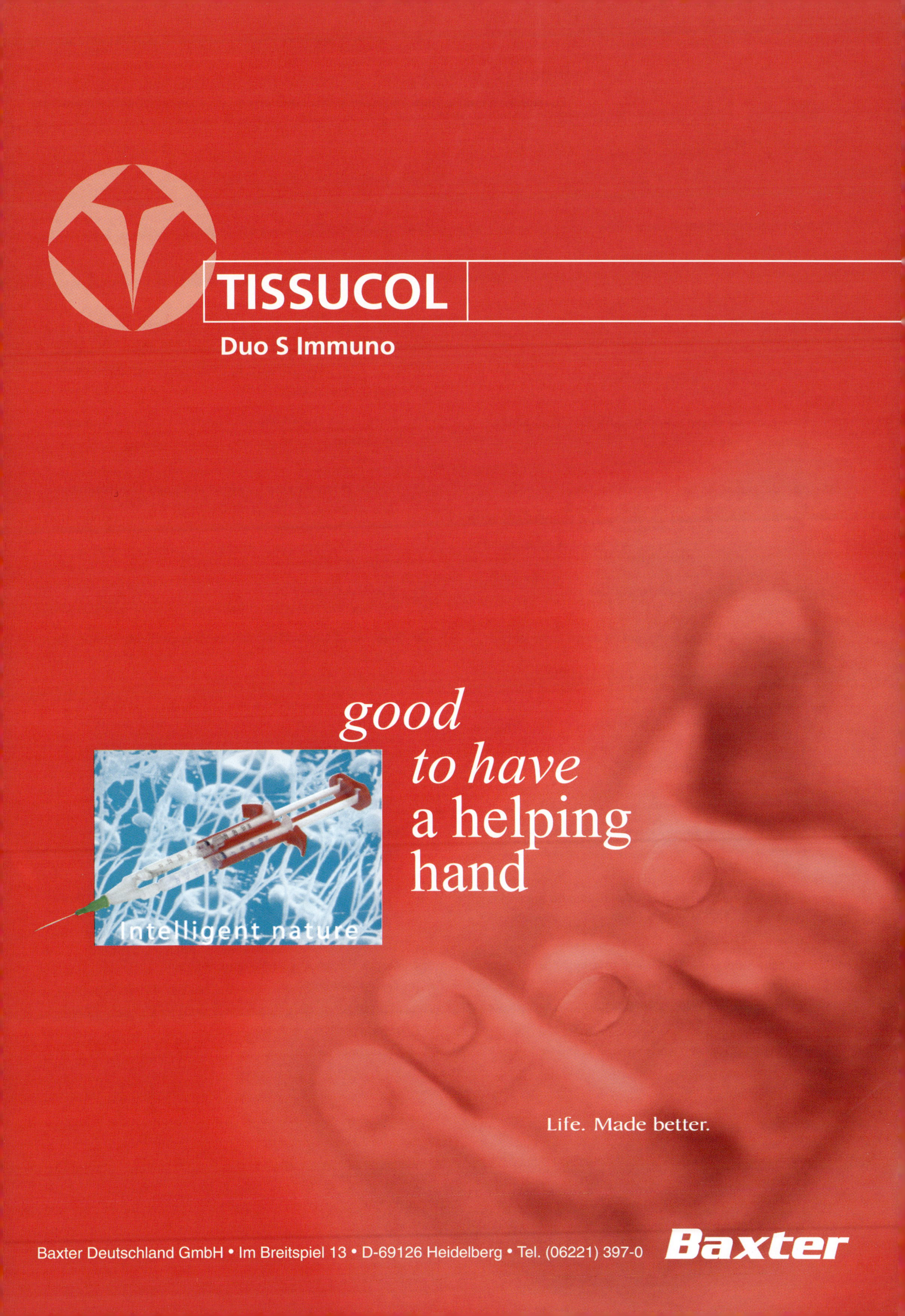
TISSUCOL
Duo S Immuno
good
to have
a helping
hand
Intelligent nature
Life. Made better.
Baxter Deutschland GmbH • Im Breitspiel 13 • D-69126 Heidelberg • Tel. (06221) 397-0
Baxter

Chirurgische Gastroenterologie Interdisziplinär

Inhalt · Contents

Band 18, Supplement 1, Juni 2002 Vol. 18, Supplement 1, June 2002

KARGER

Fax +49 761 452 07 14
E-mail Information@Karger.de
www.karger.com

Artikel (Volltext) und Inhaltsverzeichnisse sowie das vorläufige Inhaltsverzeichnis des nächsten Heftes: www.karger.com/journals/cga/cga_bk.htm

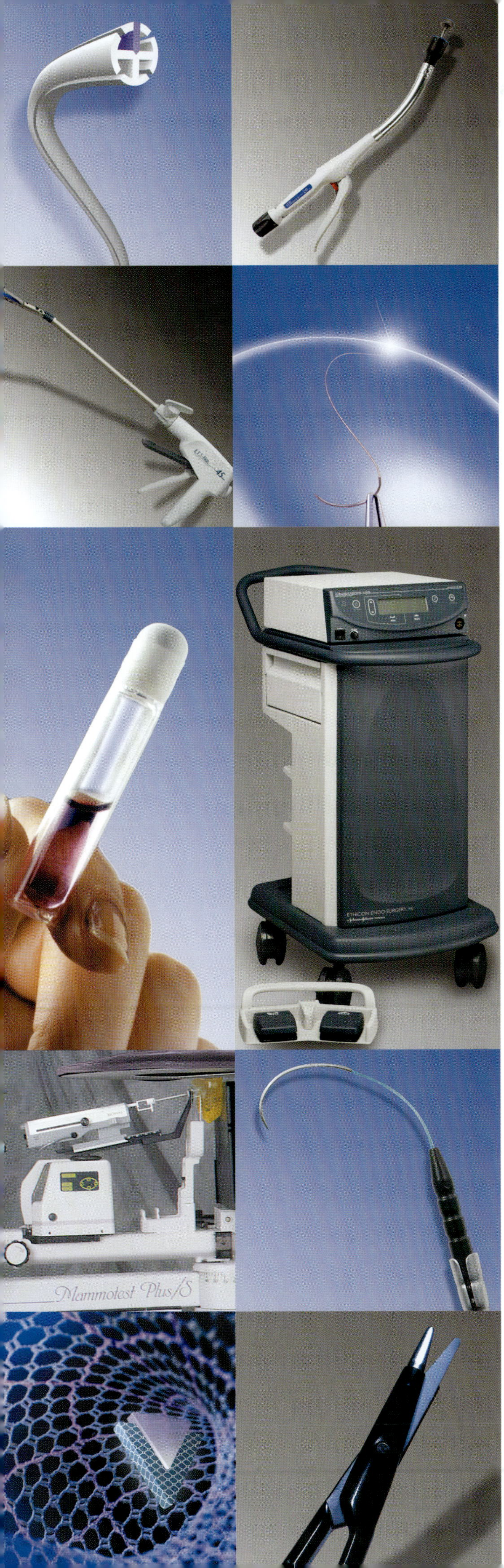
Mammotest Plus/S

Chirurgische Gastroenterologie Interdisziplinär

Chir Gastroenterol 2002;18(suppl 1):VI

Editorial

Der Spendermangel bei Organtransplantationen ist ein fortbestehendes Problem. Der Tod von bis zu 30% der Patienten auf der Warteliste zur Herz- oder Lebertransplantation macht «Die Steigerung der Organverfügbarkeit» zu einem brisanten Thema in der Transplantationsmedizin. Die zu geringe Bereitschaft zur Organspende ist nur ein Aspekt des Engpasses. Ohne Zweifel ist auf diesem Gebiet weiterhin starke Aufklärungsarbeit nötig. Ein zusätzlicher Ansatz liegt in einer besseren Motivation und der organisatorischen Unterstützung der Spenderkrankenhäuser. Als Paradigma kann unser Nachbarland Österreich gelten. Die äußerst effiziente, landesweite Organspendeorganisation in Spanien wird in einem weiteren Beitrag dargestellt. Diese Beispiele zeigen, dass mit der Ausschöpfung vorhandener Ressourcen der Organmangel reduziert werden kann. Um Schaden für unsere Patienten durch zu lange Wartezeiten bis zur Transplantation zu verhindern, wurden in den letzten Jahren auch Organe im Grenzbereich zur Transplantation akzeptiert. Dieses Vorgehen war nur auf dem Boden zunehmender Kenntnisse über Schädigungsmechanismen von Ischämie und Reperfusion sowie über Ansätze zur Protektion des Transplantats gerechtfertigt. Die nötigen Voraussetzungen zur Vergrößerung des Organpools in dieser Hinsicht ohne Gefährdung des Empfängers werden in vier Beiträgen des vorliegenden Heftes analysiert.

Ein innovativer und effizienter Ansatz zur Steigerung der Organverfügbarkeit ist die Lebendspende. Die Ausweitung des Verfahrens akzentuiert das Problem der Spendermorbidität und sogar -mortalität, besonders repräsentiert in der Transplantation des rechten Leberlappens auf erwachsene Empfänger. Dieser Brennpunkt muss deutlich machen, dass wir – getrieben von dem nicht hinzunehmenden Organmangel – einen Ausweg erarbeitet haben, der jedoch das Problem in die betroffenen Familien verlagert. Hier sind die Transplantationszentren fachübergreifend gefordert, den hohen ethischen Anforderungen in der Beratung der Betroffenen gerecht zu werden und das Verfahren mit großer Selbstkritik zu implementieren.

Vor diesem Hintergrund sollte die Organspende nach Herztod als ein weiterer Ausweg aus der Mangelsituation neu bewertet werden. Bei uns verboten, ist das Verfahren in den USA gut etabliert und führt zur Steigerung der Anzahl von Spenderorganen.

Die vorliegenden Übersichtsarbeiten orientieren sich an Plenarveranstaltungen der 10. Jahrestagung der Deutschen Transplantationsgesellschaft im November 2001 in Heidelberg. Es soll der State-of-the-Art zur Steigerung der Organverfügbarkeit aufgezeigt werden, ohne zu vergessen, dass die Verstärkung der konventionellen Organspende nach wie vor die beste Lösung darstellt.

Ernst Klar, Heidelberg

KARGER

Fax +49 761 452 07 14
E-mail Information@Karger.de
www.karger.com

Accessible online at:
www.karger.com/journals/cga

Chirurgische Gastroenterologie Interdisziplinär

Chir Gastroenterol 2002;18(suppl 1):2–4

Konventionelle Organspende: Paradigma Österreich

R. Margreiter

Klinische Abteilung für Transplantationschirurgie, Universitätsklinik für Chirurgie, Innsbruck

Transplantationsaktivitäten

In Österreich wird an den drei Universitätskliniken Wien, Graz und Innsbruck im Rahmen eigener Abteilungen Transplantationschirurgie betrieben. Weiterhin gibt es noch je ein Nierentransplantationsprogramm an zwei nichtuniversitären Kliniken in Linz. Insgesamt wurden in den Jahren 1999 und 2000 739 Nieren-, 303 Leber-, 179 Herz-, 126 Lungen-, 2 Herz-Lungen-, 60 Pankreas- sowie 8 Darm- und 2 Handtransplantationen durchgeführt (Tab. 1). Hinzu kommen noch 75 Nieren- und 10 Leberverpflanzungen von Lebendspendern. Ohne die Lebendspenden resultieren daraus 46,2 Nieren-, 18,9 Leber-, 11,2 Herz-, 7,9 Lungen- und 3,8 Pankreastransplantationen sowie 1 Darmverpflanzung pro 1 Million Einwohner und Jahr, womit sich Österreich in der Transplantationschirurgie zumindest quantitativ im weltweiten Spitzenfeld positioniert. Da das Spenderaufkommen im Jahre 1999 24,4 und 2000 23,1/1 Million Einwohner betrug, erscheint die Behauptung legitim, dass die Transplantationsaktivitäten im Lande mit eigenen Organen abgedeckt werden. Durch eine steigende Mortalität auf der Warteliste für Herz- und Lebertransplantationen und zunehmend längere Wartezeiten auf eine Nierenverpflanzung je nach Zentrum von 18–36 Monaten werden diese Erfolgsmeldungen jedoch relativiert. Dies umso mehr, wenn man bedenkt, dass Österreich in den Jahren 1990 und 1991 ein Spenderaufkommen von 29 bzw. 28/1 Million Einwohner verzeichnete, was mit einer Nierentransplantationsfrequenz von 55/1 Million Einwohner zu einer spürbaren Abnahme der Warteliste geführt hatte.

Tab. 1. Zahl der Transplantationen in den Jahren 1999 und 2000 in Österreich

Ort	Nieren		Pankreas (+ Nieren)		Leber		Herz	Lunge	Darm
	C	L			C	L			
Wien	331	47	1	(1)	151	0	110	106*	0
Graz	86	0	0		22	0	28	0	0
Innsbruck	175	21	59	(55)	130	10	41	22	8
Linz									
AOL	33	3	0		0	0	0	0	0
AOE	58	4	0		0	0	0	0	0

*2 Herz-Lungen-Transplantationen.
C = Leichenspende; L = Lebendspende; AOL = Allgemeines Krankenhaus Linz; AOE = Krankenhaus der Elisabethinen Linz.

Organspendeaktivitäten

Gesetzliche Regelung
Die Organspende ist in Österreich nicht durch ein eigenes Transplantationsgesetz, sondern seit dem 18. Juni 1982 im Rahmen des Landes-Krankenanstaltengesetzes geregelt und entspricht der so genannten Widerspruchslösung. So heißt es im § 62 a (1): «Die Entnahme ist unzulässig, wenn den Ärzten eine Erklärung vorliegt, mit der der Verstorbene oder, vor dessen Tod, sein gesetzlicher Vertreter eine Organspende ausdrücklich abgelehnt hat. Die Entnahme darf nicht zu einer die Pietät verletzenden Verunstaltung der Leiche führen.» Nicht explizit geregelt ist hingegen die Entnahme von Organen oder Geweben von Lebenden, wobei bestehende allgemeine Rechtsgrundsätze den Transplantationschirurgen ausreichende Rechtssicherheit bieten. Dass diese Art der gesetzlichen Regelung von breiten Kreisen der Bevölkerung mitgetragen wird, mag darin begründet sein, dass Autopsien von Patienten, die in öffentlichen Krankenanstalten verstorben sind, nicht nur auf sanitätspolizeilichen oder gerichtlichen Antrag, sondern auch zur Wahrung wissenschaftlichen Interesses, insbesondere bei diagnostischen Unklarheiten, seit über 200 Jahren gesetzlich (Krankenanstaltengesetz § 25) vorgeschrieben sind und sich deshalb die Bevölkerung an die Vorstellung der postmortalen Leichenöffnung offenbar gewöhnt hat. Kritisiert wurde nicht nur im Inland lediglich das Fehlen einer zentralen Registrierungsstelle zur Hinterlegung des Widerspruchs. Dieser Mangel wurde zwischenzeitlich behoben.
Um dem rückläufigen Spenderaufkommen im letzten Jahrzehnt Rechnung zu tragen, wurde im Krankenanstaltengesetzt § 59 d (1) festgeschrieben: «Der Strukturfond hat die Mittel zur Förderung des Transplantationswesens zur Erreichung folgender Ziele einzusetzen: 1. Im Bereiche der Organtransplantationen ist die Konti-

KARGER

Fax +49 761 452 07 14
E-mail Information@Karger.de
www.karger.com

Accessible online at:
www.karger.com/journals/cga

Prof. Dr. R. Margreiter
Klinische Abteilung für Transplantationschirurgie
Universitätsklinik für Chirurgie
Anichstraße 35
A-6020 Innsbruck (Österreich)
Te. +43 512 504 0

nuität im Spenderaufkommen auf hohem Niveau (etwa 30 Organspender/1 Million Einwohner) sicherzustellen.» Dieses Gesetz wurde erst unlängst beschlossen, weshalb seine Wirksamkeit noch nicht belegt werden kann. Es sollte sich jedoch den Krankhausträgern gegenüber als durchaus wirksames Argument erweisen.

Organisation

Bestanden bis vor 10 Jahren in Österreich für das Organspendewesen keinerlei Organisationsstrukturen, so wurde vor genau einem Jahrzehnt eine Institution ins Leben gerufen, die das Transplantationswesen in Österreich koordinieren und unterstützen sollte. Diese Institution ist innerhalb des Österreichischen Bundesinstituts für Gesundheitswesen (ÖBIG) angesiedelt. Bei dem ÖBIG wiederum handelt es sich um eine selbstständige Einrichtung, die das Gesundheitsministerium in wesentlichen Fragen des Gesundheitswesens, vor allem hinsichtlich des Bedarfs an stationären Einrichtungen, berät. Zu den Aufgaben des ÖBIG-Transplant gehören:

- Förderung des Organ- und Gewebeaufkommens
- Förderung des Informations- und Datenaustauschs
- Öffentlichkeitsarbeit
- Dokumentation des Transplantationsgeschehens in Österreich
- Erstellung von Analysen und Durchführung von Planungsarbeiten als Grundlagen für die Verhandlungsführung von Entscheidungsträgern im Transplantationsgeschehen
- Führung des Widerspruchregisters gegen Organspende.

Die Organisationsstrukturen des ÖBIG-Transplant sind in Abbildung 1 dargestellt.

Stand man dieser halbstaatlichen Einrichtung von ärztlicher Seite anfänglich skeptisch gegenüber, hat sie sich doch bisher als sehr segensreich erwiesen. So gelang es ihr relativ schnell, eine bis dahin nicht existierende kostendeckende Aufwandentschädigung für die Leistungen im Zusammenhang mit der Organentnahme zu erwirken und nachhaltig sicherzustellen. Zum anderen wurde ein Widerspruchsregister etabliert und geführt. Darüber hinaus vergibt das ÖBIG Geldmittel für die Strukturverbesserung der Transplantationszentren. Installiert wurden auch so genannte Transplantationsbeauftragte an allen potenziellen Spenderkrankenhäusern. Diese mussten von der ärztlichen Krankenhausleitung namhaft gemacht werden. Zu ihren Aufgaben zählt das Bemühen um das Spenderaufkommen vor Ort. Vor etwa einem Jahr wurde Österreich in vier Spenderregionen gegliedert, wobei Südtirol seit Jahren offiziell vom Transplantationszentrum Innsbruck betreut wird (Abb. 2). Organe aus Bundesländern ohne eigene Transplantationsprogramme werden entsprechend der Zahl der Patienten auf der Warteliste bzw. der letztjährigen Aktivitäten der einzelnen Transplantationszentren für das Spenderbundesland zugeteilt. Zur Betreuung dieser Spenderregionen wurde vorerst nur für die Region Nord ein so genannter Transplantationsreferent ernannt. Dabei handelt es sich um den Leiter einer großen Abteilung für Anästhesiologie und Intensivpflege einer neurochirurgischen Klinik. Ihm gelang im ersten Jahr seiner Tätigkeit eine signifikante Steigerung der Zahl der Organspender in seiner Region. Die Ernennung von Transplantationsbeauftragten für die drei anderen Regionen wird zur Zeit vorbereitet. Von unserer Bundeshauptstadt abgesehen, ist die Zahl an Transplantationskoordinatoren in unserem Lande im internationalen Vergleich als gering zu bezeichnen und entspricht nicht ganz den Aktivitäten der einzelnen Zentren: So verfügt Wien über insgesamt sechs Koordinatoren, Innsbruck über zwei und Graz über eine Stelle, während Linz ohne Koordinator auskommen muss.

Diskussion

Trotz aller dieser Initiativen ist es in den letzten Jahren nicht zu der erhofften Steigerung der Zahl der Organspender gekommen, obwohl wir wissen, dass ausreichend Spender vorhanden wären. Über die möglichen Ursachen kann teilweise nur spekuliert werden. Tatsache ist, dass die Zahl tödlicher Verkehrsunfälle in den letzten Jahren wohl zurückgegangen ist, dies jedoch sicherlich nicht in dem Maße wie die Zahl der Organspender. Andererseits hat die Zahl fataler Sport- und Freizeitunfälle im gleichen Zeitraum erheblich zugenommen. Entscheidend scheint mir zu sein, dass Identifikation und Konditionierung beileibe nicht an allen Krankenhäusern zu den selbstverständlichen Aufgaben gehören,

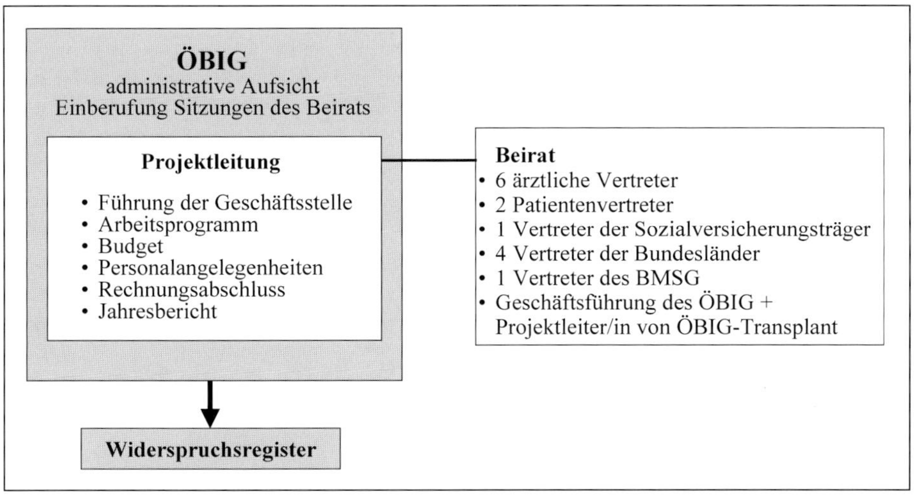

Abb. 1. Organisationsstruktur des ÖBIG-Transplant.

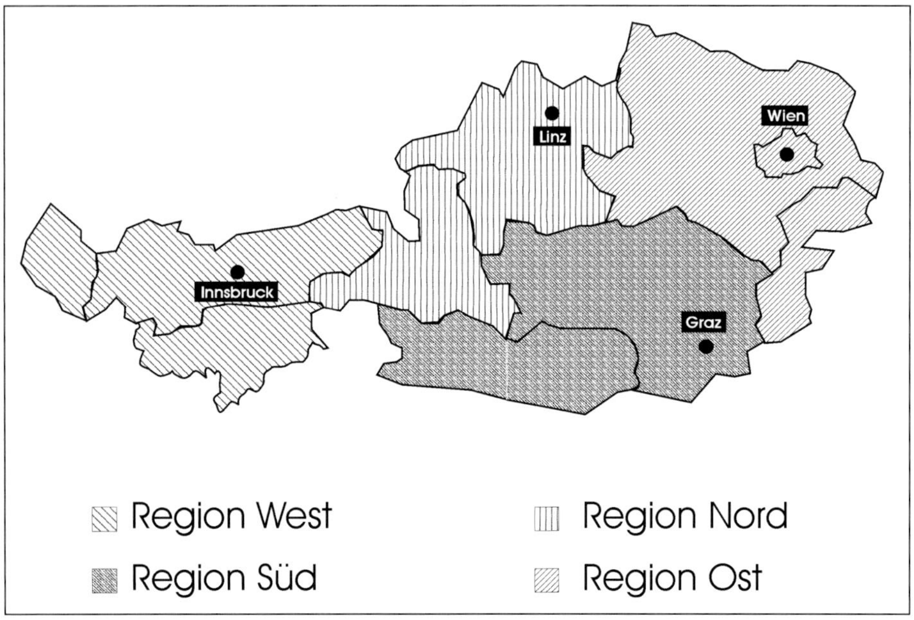

Abb. 2. Spenderregionen in Österreich.

sondern weitestgehend von der Einstellung der für die betreffende Intensivpflegestation verantwortlichen Ärzte und zum Teil auch des Pflegepersonals abhängen. Im Gegensatz zu Spanien gibt es keine regelmäßige Besprechungen zwischen der lokalen Ärzteschaft und Vertretern der Transplantationsmedizin bzw. der Gesundheitsbehörde. Zudem besteht keine Berichtspflicht, weder für die Krankenanstalten noch die Transplantationsbeauftragten, sodass der Installation dieser Transplantationsbeauftragten ein Alibicharakter zukommt. Hinsichtlich der Ausstattung der österreichischen Transplantationszentren mit Koordinatoren besteht Nachbesserungsbedarf. Es ist durchaus vorstellbar, dass eine Aufstockung der Zahl an Koordinatoren sich positiv auf das Spenderaufkommen auswirkt. Nur am Rande sei erwähnt, dass die direkt an die Krankenhäuser geleistete finanzielle Abgeltung von Leistungen im Zusammenhang mit Organspenden mit der Begründung, dass diese ohnehin von Diensthabenden erbracht würden, nicht an die Leistungsträger weitergegeben werden, was für diese sicherlich keinen Anreiz darstellen dürfte. Nicht unerwähnt darf bleiben, dass in fast allen Spenderkrankenhäusern trotz der bestehenden Rechtslage die Zustimmungs-, zumindest jedoch die Informationslösung praktiziert wird. Dies hat wohl zu einer minimal höheren Ablehnungsrate – genaue Zahlen liegen nicht vor – geführt, wurde jedoch besonders vom Pflegepersonal sehr positiv aufgenommen. Da in Spanien in gleicher Weise vorgegangen wird, scheint damit belegt zu sein, dass die rechtliche Regelung der Organspende wesentlich geringeren Einfluss auf das Spenderaufkommen hat als vielfach angenommen.

Zusammenfassung

Spenderzahlen und in direkter Abhängigkeit die Transplantationsaktivitäten in Österreich gehören mit zu den höchsten weltweit. Die steigende Zahl der Todesfälle auf der Warteliste für vitale Organe sowie die noch zu langen Wartezeiten auf eine Nierenverpflanzung machen jedoch den Mangel an Spenderorganen auch in unserem Lande deutlich. Eine Problemlösung erscheint mir nur dadurch möglich, dass – eventuell auch durch Druck von Seiten der Öffentlichkeit – Spenderidentifikation und Betreuung von den zuständigen Einrichtungen nicht mehr als freiwillige Zusatzleistung, sondern als integraler Bestandteil des Aufgabenkatalogs einer jeden Intensivpflegeeinheit verstanden und damit zur Selbstverständlichkeit und Normalität wird.

Subskriptions-Angebot:
EUR 39.90/CHF 60.–

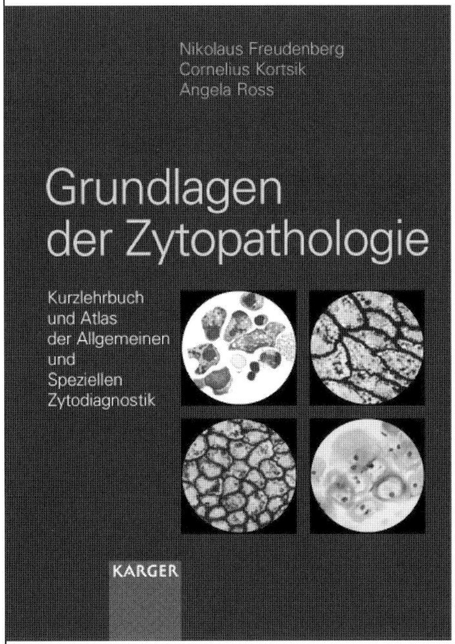

Nikolaus Freudenberg (Freiburg)
Cornelius Kortsik (Mainz)
Angela Ross (Freiburg)

Grundlagen der Zytopathologie

Kurzlehrbuch und Atlas der allgemeinen und speziellen Zytodiagnostik

Endokrinologie, Gynäkologie, Innere Medizin, Krankenpflege, Medizinische Technik, Onkologie, Pathologie, Pneumologie, Radiologie, Zytologie

Aus dem Inhalt:

Allgemeiner Teil
I. Zytologische Methoden
II. Allgemeine Zytologie
III. Allgemeine Zytopathologie
1. Funktionsverlust
2. Funktionssteigerung
3. Dysfunktion
4. Grundlagen der Zytodiagnostik

Spezieller Teil
I. Respirationstrakt
II. Ergüsse der serösen Körperhöhlen
III. Cervix uteri
IV. Mamma
V. Schilddrüse

Kompetente Autoren, brillante Farbabbildungen und fachkundige Erklärungen machen dieses Buch zu einem Standardwerk für die Ausbildung in diagnostischer Zytologie!

Im ersten Kapitel werden die methodischen Grundlagen zur Gewinnung, Bearbeitung und Auswertung von zytologischem Material beschrieben. Es werden die Techniken der Exfoliativ- und Punktionszytologie, des Ausstreichens und des Zellblocks dargestellt sowie die verschiedenen Fixierungsverfahren, zytologische Standardfärbungen und Spezialfärbungen. Ausserdem werden die Techniken der Enzym- und Immunzytochemie und die Auswertungsmöglichkeiten erklärt.

In den Kapiteln über allgemeine Zytopathologie werden die verschiedenen, diagnostisch relevanten Reaktionsmuster der Zelle systematisch abgehandelt und in den zytodiagnostischen Zusammenhang gebracht. Die Fragen der Aktivierung, Hypertrophie und Hyperplasie wie auch die Problematik der Degeneration bis hin zum Zelltod (Nekrose, Onkose, Apoptose) werden an praktischen Beispielen von Entzündung, Immunantwort und regressiven Veränderungen erklärt. An zytologischen Beispielen werden die Begriffe Metaplasie, Parakeratose, Dyskeratose und Regeneratepithel und deren biologische Bedeutung erläutert. Weiterhin werden die neuesten Erkenntnisse zur Onkogenese und deren Folgen für die prognostischen Aussagen der Zytodiagnostik an Dysplasie- und Tumorzellen dargelegt.

Die Kapitel über spezielle Zytopathologie behandeln systematisch die Zytologie und Zytopathologie häufiger, zytodiagnostisch erfassbarer Organkrankheiten des Respirationstrakts, der Ergüsse in den serösen Körperhöhlen, der Cervix uteri, der Mamma und der Schilddrüse.

KI 01236_SKD

www.karger.com

Freudenberg, N. (Freiburg); Kortsik, C. (Mainz); Ross, A. (Freiburg)
Grundlagen der Zytopathologie
Kurzlehrbuch und Atlas der allgemeinen und speziellen Zytodiagnostik
ca. 140 S., ca. 280 Abb. (grösstenteils vierfarbig)
Erscheinungstermin: 2. Quartal 2002
voraussichtlicher Ladenpreis: EUR 49.90 / CHF 76.–
Subskriptionspreis: EUR 39.90 / CHF 60.–
Preisänderungen vorbehalten
EUR-Preise nur für Deutschland
ISBN 3–8055–7255–7

KARGER

Bestellformular

Bitte senden Sie: ____ Expl.
Bei Vorauszahlung Porto und Verpackung zu Lasten des Verlags

Ich bezahle:
☐ Mit Scheck ☐ Nach Erhalt der Rechnung
Bitte belasten Sie diese Bestellung meiner Kreditkarte
☐ American Express ☐ Diners ☐ Eurocard
☐ MasterCard ☐ Visa

Kreditkarten-Nr.: ____________________

Gültig bis: ____________________

Senden Sie Ihre Bestellung an Ihre Buchhandlung, Agentur, direkt an den Verlag oder an eine seiner Vertretungen.

Fax: +49 761 45 207 14
S. Karger GmbH, Postfach, D–79095 Freiburg (Deutschland)
E-Mail information@karger.de, **www.karger.com**

Name/Adresse: ____________________

____

____

____

____

Datum: ____________________

Unterschrift: ____________________

Chirurgische Gastroenterologie Interdisziplinär

Chir Gastroenterol 2002;18(suppl 1):7–16

The Spanish Organizational Structure for Organ Donation – Up to Date

B. Miranda J. Cañón N. Cuende

Organización Nacional de Trasplantes, Madrid, Spain

Summary

At the end of 1989, the Organización Nacional de Trasplantes (ONT) was created within the Spanish Department of Health. It has become a common meeting place for professionals involved in all types of transplantation, the central and autonomous administrations, the media, and Spanish society in general. It has a formal but flexible management structure, which ensures that the hospital transplant coordinators working at the grass-roots level have a sense of involvement and are accountable for performance. These coordinators are responsible for the process of organ donation and procurement within hospitals. The ONT deals with organ sharing and management of waiting lists, arranges for transplant teams or organ transport, maintains the official statistics on organ donation and transplantation activity, and keeps interested groups informed. The ONT is concerned with training programs and research in the field of organ donation and transplantation. It is the unit in charge of official reports in this field, and it guarantees the complete equity and transparency of the system. Within this framework, the average annual rate of solid-organ donations increased from 14 donors per million population (pmp) in 1989 to 34 donors pmp in June 2000. The average age of donors has increased year after year, and more than 30% of current donors are older than 60 years. Most donors (75%) now die of cerebrovascular incidents, and only 21% die in car accidents (in 1992, 43% died in car accidents). In Spain, the current rate of family refusal of donation is 21.5%, a decrease from the 30% rate seen in the early 1990s. All of these changes are the result of efforts to overcome various obstacles, such as untrained or undertrained staff, unidentified donors, and reluctance to approach grieving families. This means the professionalization of organ donation together with an organization focusing on the promotion and facilitation of all these actions. Coordinators are identifying more and more potential in all types of hospitals, stating that the problem is not only a lack of donors but rather a failure to convert potential into actual. Overall, analysis of the organ donation process, detecting the circumstantial obstacles in the different hospitals or regions, provides with the means to find the most appropriate solutions.

Zusammenfassung

Am Jahresende 1989 wurde die «Organización Nacional de Trasplantes» (ONT) innerhalb der Spanischen Gesundheitsbehörde ins Leben gerufen. Die ONT dient inzwischen als Einrichtung zum Informationsaustausch für Spezialisten in der Transplantation, für zentrale und autonome Verwaltungsbehörden und ist zugleich Ansprechpartner für die Medien und für die spanische Gesellschaft. Die ONT hat eine formelle, aber flexible Managementstruktur, wodurch sichergestellt wird, dass die an der Basis arbeitenden Transplantationskoordinatoren direkt involviert sind. Sie tragen insbesondere für den Prozess der Organspende und -beschaffung innerhalb der Krankenhäuser die Verantwortung. Die ONT befasst sich mit Organverteilung und mit der Führung von Wartelisten, organisiert Transplantations-Teams und den Organtransport, erstellt die offizielle Statistik über Organspenden und Transplantationsaktivitäten und informiert interessierte Kreise. Sie kümmert sich um Trainingsprogramme und Forschung im Bereich Organspende und Transplantation, hat die Verantwortung für offizielle Berichte aus diesem Bereich und garantiert völlige Unparteilichkeit und Transparenz des Systems. In diesem Rahmen wuchs die durchschnittliche jährliche Organspenderate von 14 Spendern pro 1 Million Einwohner (pME) im Jahr 1989 auf 34 Spender pME im Juni 2000. Das durchschnittliche Alter der Spender stieg jährlich auf ein jetziges Spenderalter über 60 Jahren in mehr als 30% der Fälle. Die meisten Spender (75%) sterben derzeit infolge eines zerebrovaskulären Geschehens, nur 21% sterben bei einem Autounfall (1992 waren es noch 43%). In Spanien besteht derzeit eine Verweigerungsrate zur Organspende von Seiten der Familien von 21,5%; in den frühen 1990er Jahren waren es noch 30%. Diese Veränderungen sind das Ergebnis von Bemühungen, diverse Hindernisse – wie untrainiertes oder zu wenig trainiertes Personal, nicht identifizierte Spender sowie das Widerstreben, sich mit trauernden Familien zu befassen – zu überwinden. Das bedeutet die Professionalisierung der Organspende in Verbindung mit einer Organisation, die sich auf die Promotion und Förderung all dieser Aktionen konzentriert. Koordinatoren identifizieren zunehmend mehr Potenzial in allen Krankenhäusern. Es sei nicht nur ein Spendermangel, sondern auch das Versäumnis, Potenzial in Realität umzusetzen. Allgemein erleichtert die Analyse des Organspendeprozesses das Erkennen und Überwinden von Hindernissen in verschiedenen Krankenhäusern und Regionen.

(Übersetzung/Bearbeitung: Dr. P. Schemmer
Chirurgische Universitätsklinik Heidelberg)

KARGER

Fax +49 761 452 07 14
E-mail Information@Karger.de
www.karger.com

Accessible online at:
www.karger.com/journals/cga

Dr. B. Miranda
Organización Nacional de Trasplantes
c/ Sinesio Delgado, 8
E-28029 Madrid (Spain)
Tel. +34 91 314-2406, Fax -2969/56
E-mail bmiranda@msc.es

Introduction

Spanish transplantation history started in 1965 with the first kidney transplants performed in Madrid and Barcelone. In 1979 we got the transplant law, hence transplantation activity using cadaveric kidneys steadily increased during the early 1980s, and heart and liver transplantation programs were started in the middle of the decade. After a peak of 16 donors per million population (pmp) and 1,182 kidney grafts in 1986, the figures decreased by 20% in 1987, and the annual number of kidneys available for transplantation hovered around 1,000 in 1987, 1988, and 1989. This led to exponential growth of the waiting list. As a consequence, a censure was lodged with the kidney patients' associations and the Ombudsman intervened. This, together with the increasing complexity of heart and liver transplantation procedures, waiting list management, and other organizational tasks led to the decision of the Ministry of Health to set up the ONT.

The Organization: General Characteristics

Spain is a European Community country with a population of 41.1 million people living in 17 autonomous regions. The National Health System (NHS) is composed of all of the facilities and public services devoted to health. Today, public health assistance is available for 99.4% of the population, the budget for Health Services being 6% of the Inner product. The health counsellors from each Autonomous Region form the Interterritorial Council for the National Health System, which is presided over by the Minister of Health and Consumer Affairs and is in charge of the coordination of health policies. This Council has different permanent working groups, one of these being the Transplantation Group.

Legal Aspects

Legal statements for organ and tissue donation and transplantation are included in 3 main legal texts [1–3]:

1. Ley de Trasplantes – 1979.
2. Real Decreto de extracción e implante de tejidos y células para trasplante – 1996.
3. Real Decreto de extracción e implante de órganos para trasplante – 1999.

They cover all main points requiring legal support:
- Diagnosis and certification of death.
- Consent for donation.
- Criteria for official authorization for organ retrieval and transplantation.
- Confidentiality of data.
- Removal – management – processing transport – storage and grafting of organs, cells and tissues.
- Traceability of donors and recipients.
- Need of avoiding, pursuing and denouncing any form of organ trade.
- Coordination of activities.
- The transplantation law is technically similar to the corresponding laws in other Western countries:
- Death is defined as the total and irreversible cessation of brain or cardiorespiratory functions and must be certified by 3 doctors in case of brain death. Clinical evaluation and complementary tests needed to declare the death are detailed within the legal texts.
- Organs and tissues may be retrieved only after obtaining the consent from the donor or the donor's family.
- It is clearly stated that no compensation may be paid either. Either for donation or for grafted organs.

The ONT as a Supportive System for Organ Donation and Transplantation Procedures

Organ donation and transplantation procedures are large and complex, involving more than 100 professionals (both health care and non-health care workers) and requiring more than 20 hours of continuous work. These procedures are probably the only medical activity that cannot be done with only technical and economic resources but need the direct involvement of society (fig. 1). Moreover, in any country, the organs available for transplantation are matching the demand, leading to the possibility of either negative or positive deviations that need to be avoided.

The ONT then emphasized the need of a network of professionals who would be responsible for organ donation as a whole covering all aspects and working at all levels: the national level, the regional level, and the hospital level. This meant the professionalization of organ donation and implied the need for training and organizational support.

These professionals, so-called transplant coordinators working at the grass-roots level, must have a sense of involvement and are accountable for performance [4]. Most coordinators are qualified physicians, primarily intensive care specialists or nephrologists, who work part-time on transplant coordinating tasks (table 1). Their main aim is organ procurement, and they are responsible for all the entire process of procurement (fig. 1). Spain currently has 139 hospital-coordinating teams, one in each hospital, that are officially authorized to develop donation and organ procurement processes.

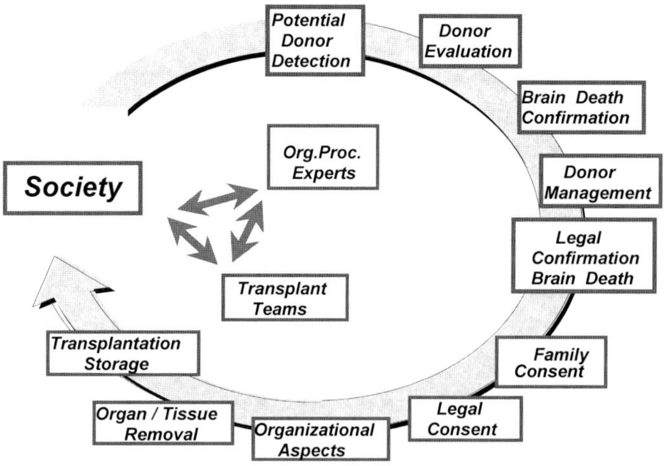

Fig. 1. The process of organ donation and transplantation.

Table 1. Characteristics of hospital-based transplant coordinators[1]

Qualification	Physicians and nurses
Dedication	Part time
Report to	Medical Director
Background	Intensive Care – Nephrology
Location	Within the hospital staff
Main aim	Organ procurement
Increasingly involved in:	Logistics of organ procurement and transplantation
	Education programs
	Resource management
	Relations with media

[1] ONT central office and regional transplant coordinators act as a service agency supporting all the processes.

In many hospitals, transplant coordinator teams are formed by one single person working part time, but when activity is bigger enough or the hospital includes different transplant programs, a group of physicians and nurses forms the transplant coordinating team.

The Transplant Committee of the Interregional Council, on which all autonomous communities are represented by the regional transplant coordinators, is responsible for discussing and drawing up the various policies that affect organ, tissue and bone marrow procurement and transplantation. The central office for ONT acts as the secretariat of this Interregional Council, and the National Coordinator usually presides over it. Every year, among many other things, this Committee discusses organ allocation criteria within itself and with the transplant teams, and these criteria are modified according to the previous year's results to avoid positive or negative deviations. Variables, such as primary disease, code of urgency, blood group, age and weight, or city of residence, are analyzed to ensure that every group of patients has the same chance of getting an organ [5].

The central office of ONT acts as a Service Agency supporting all the system and deals with organ sharing and management of waiting lists. It arranges for transplant teams and organ shifts. It maintains official statistics and reports on organ donation and transplantation activity, keeping informed all interested groups. It maintains continuously systems to address any doubt or questions about organ procurement and transplantation through a 24-hour telephone line and an active web site. ONT is concerned with training programs and research in the field of organ donation and transplantation. It tries to be a common form for debate in any field related to organ donation or transplantation.

Differences to Other Systems

Most coordinating systems worldwide are dedicated to maintain and control waiting lists; to organ sharing; to maintain statistics; and in some instances, to organ or team shift arrangements [6]. Nevertheless, we strongly believe that the coordinating system should fulfil two fundamental missions: It should support the entire process, and it should perform all of the organizational tasks that organ sharing and waiting list management entails.

There seems to be general agreement about the need for some kind of 'suprahospital' organization to support transplantation activities. Such organizations are quite different from country to country and can be structured in different combinations. Ours can be defined as follows (*marked):

– **Scope:**	Regional
	* National
	Supranational
– **Size:**	Small: < 10 million inhabitants
	* Medium: > 10 million and < 60 million inhabitants
	Large: > 60 million inhabitants
– **Reporting to:**	Professionals
	* Health Authorities
	Mixed
– **Structure:**	Non-profit Foundation
	Private agency
	* State agency
– **Budget:**	Hospitals
	* Health Department
	Companies
	Mixed
– **General philosophy:**	Centralized
	* Decentralized
– **Competences:**	* Organ sharing
	* Organ procurement
	* Promotion of donation
– **Activities:**	* Solid organs
	* Hemopoietic Progenitors
	* Tissues, cells

The differences among organizations result from their origins and histories, their health systems and the resources, and the personal profiles of the founders and directors. We have little doubt that the ideal situation is an integrated approach, supporting the entire process of organ donation, procurement, distribution, and grafting. The organization should be aware of data and, thus, be able to detect problems, promote the most appropriate solutions, and participate in research and training. It must also be responsible for ensuring transparency and equity.

An apparent contradiction has been pointed out. It is accepted that the larger the donor pool, the better the match [7]. Urgent patients and difficult recipients (i.e., children and highly sensitized patients) cannot be treated efficiently within the scope of a small organization. However, many data also support the idea that smaller organizations are more efficient than larger ones [8]. Big, centralized organizations that do not allow full participation in the decision-making process are very unmotivating. A decentralized system formed by 1) local organizations that focus mainly on organ procurement and promotion of donation and 2) large structures that focus on promoting organ sharing and cooperation seems to be the most effective.

In any case, organ donation and distribution are fully in the responsibility of health administrations, and these administrations should be obliged to provide the necessary resources and guarantee the fairness, transparency, and safety of the whole system [9].

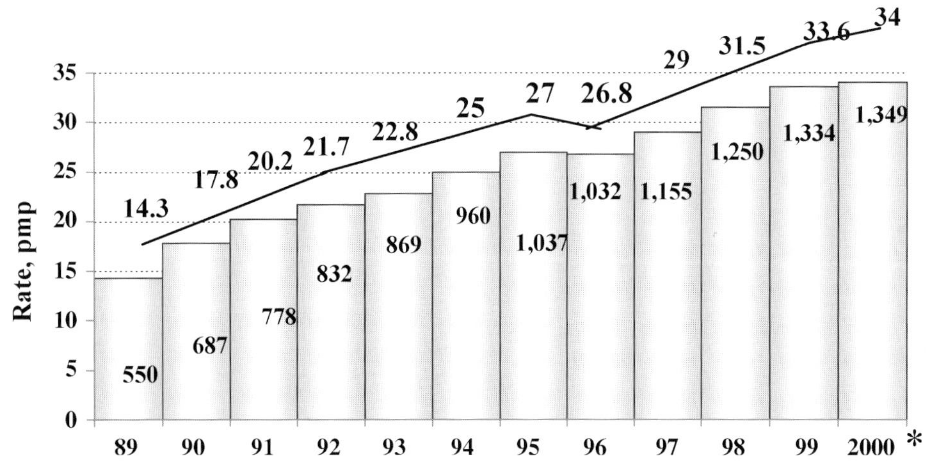

Fig. 2. Evolution of organ donation in Spain. Total numbers (depicted *in* the bars) and annual rates pmp (above the bars). Interannual rate June 30, 1999 to June 30, 2000.

Organ and Tissue Procurement Budget

There is no doubt nowadays about clinical benefits of organ and tissue transplantation, not only in what refers to survival rates [10, 11] but also in terms of quality of life [12]. It is clearly admitted that transplantation is a therapeutic option that must be offered to the patients who could benefit. There is no Health Department doubting about the need of investing in transplantation units, being even a sign of quality standard for the hospitals in which they are located. In Spain, transplantation processes have an annual general budget over EUR 152,000,000. Nevertheless, it is well known that the main obstacle for the full development of organ donation and transplantation is the number of available organs and not exactly the economical limits, hence the need of improving the number of organ donors [13]. It must be well understood, as well, that organ donation is a hospital medical activity, as any other medical activity, and so far needs its own financial support. It can never be an overload (either in terms of work or money) for other units within the hospital. Organ and tissue donation deserves special personnel and financing in order not to interfere with the normal life of the hospital. All hospitals officially authorized to maintain organ procurement programs got a specific budget for that. Same way the national and regional offices as well as the training programs or research activities in the field of organ donation deserves financial support.

All budget for the network dedicated to organ procurement each year is around EUR 15,000,000 (means less than 10% of the budget that covers transplantation activities). This figure includes the extra-salary for the transplant coordinating teams and surgical teams for removal, as well as any test or evaluation for the donor, cost of the day/bed, etc. Also it covers global administration and training courses costs. The payment model for the extrawork done by the coordinating and surgical teams is different depending on the Region and it could be fixed, depending on the activity or in a mixed way.

The Annual Budget (EUR) is divided as follows:

Hospital-based costs	10,000,000
Regional administrative and promotional programs	2,000,000
National office	1,800,000
Training programs	600,000

Evolution of Organ Donation and Transplantation

Since the basic personnel infrastructure was developed in 1990, the number of solid-organ donors has increased steadily (fig. 2). The average current annual rate is 34 donors pmp. Not only the number of donors but the number of organs retrieved has increased considerably; the percentage of multiorgan donor retrievals soared from 30% in 1989 to 85% in 1994, maintained up to now. We have noted important variations in the characteristics of these solid-organ donors. Their average age has increased year after year, resulting in a difference of more than 10 years of age between donors in 1992 and donors in 2000 (38 ± 12 to 49 ± 13). More than 30% of our current donors are older than 60 years, and more than 11% are older than 70 years (fig. 3). Traditionally, the most common source of po-

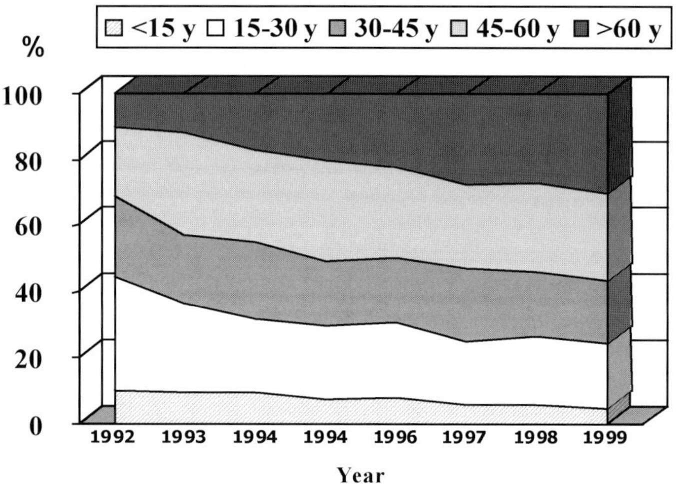

Fig. 3. Age groups among organ donors in Spain, 1992–2000.

Age group, years	1992	1993	1994	1995	1996	1997	1998	1999
>60	10	11.5	17	20.5	22	28	27	30.3
45–60	21	31.5	28	30	27.6	25.8	27.1	26.5
30–45	25	20.5	23	20	19.8	21.9	19.4	19.2
15–30	34	27	23	22.5	22.8	19.5	20.5	19.6
<15	10	9.5	9	7	7.7	5.8	5.7	4.4

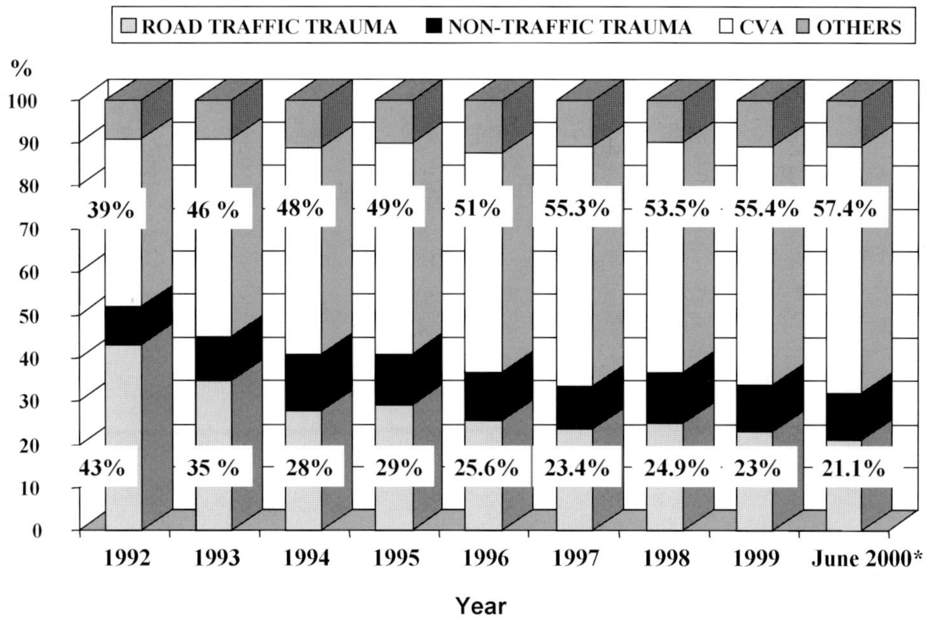

Fig. 4. Cause of death of organ donors in Spain, 1992–2000. CVA = Cerebrovascular accident. June 1999 to June 2000.

tential donations was cranial trauma patients, but Spain has seen a reversal in the percentage of deaths caused by trauma and cerebrovascular accidents (fig. 4). These changes are directly related with a 40% decrease in the number of fatal traffic accidents since 1991, and an important increase in other types of donor identification allowed the continuous rise in donor rate.

These changes in the donors' characteristics also led to an increase in the number of organs discarded once procured and examined. In fact, no solid organ from 76 donors in 1997, 88 in 1998, 117 in 1999 and 60 between January and June 2000 could be used after the retrieval due to a lack of recipient or to histological findings. The detailed analysis for kidney retrieval and transplantation gives us some important information (table 2). One could think that very old donors, with diabetic or hypertensive antecedents, should not be considered for surgical and histological evaluation. Nevertheless, we think that all potential donors should be taken into account; it is better to discard after a careful evaluation than not to have any possibility of discard or graft because we have already discarded those organs a priori.

Table 2. Kidney retrieval and transplantation in Spain, 1999

Kidney donors	Kidneys used			p
	none	one	both	
Number	197	159	933	
Age, years	60.8 ± 15	51.3 ± 19	42 ± 18	< 0.0001
Cause of death				
Trauma, %	15.3	23	40	< 0.005
ACV, %	73.7	66	49	
Other, %	11	11	11	
Hypertension (known)				
Yes, %	58.00	41	21	< 0.005
No, %	42.00	59	79	
n (data available)	137	121	674	
Diabetes (known)				
Yes, %	18.4	12	5.8	< 0.005
No, %	81.6	88	94.2	
n (data available)	103	100	606	

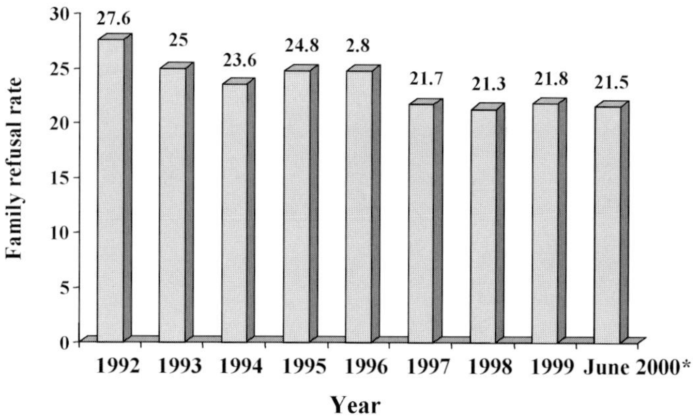

Fig. 5. Family refusal rate. Spain, 1992–1999. * June 1999 to June 2000.

The approach to the donor's family is very sensitive and is a key point, because it relates to the human drama represented by death. In Spain, the rate of family refusal of transplantation decreased from 27.6% of all interviews for donation in 1992 to 21.7% in 1999 (404 refusals among 1.849 interviews) (fig. 5). During the first 5 months of 2000, the rate of family refusal has remained stable at 21.5%.

Table 3 shows the evolution of the overall activity in solid-organ transplantation over the past few years in Spain.

Are We Meeting the Needs for Organ Transplantation?

The continuous increase in the availability of organs (and, consequently, in the number of kidney transplants) together with the maintenance of the prevalence and incidence of chronic renal fail-

Table 3. Transplantation activity

	Year											
	1989	1990	1991*	1992*	1993*	1994	1995	1996	1997	1998	1999	2000*
Cadaveric donors												
n	569	681	778	832	869	960	1,037	1,032	1,155	1,250	1,334	1,349
pmp	14	17.7	20.2	21.7	22.6	25	7	26.8	29	31.5	33.6	34
Multiorgan donors, %	30	51	64	69	70.5	77	83	79.5	82.3	84.5	85.3	85
Cadaveric kidney transplants												
n	1,021	1,224	1,355	1,477	1,473	1,613	1,765	1,685	1,841	1,976	2,006	2,007
pmp	26.5	31.8	35.2	38.4	38.4	42	46	43.8	46.6	49.8	50.6	50.6
Living related kidney transplants												
n	18	16	16	15	15	20	35	22	20	19	17	
pmp	0.5	0.4	0.4	0.4	0.4	0.5	0.9	1.3	0.5	0.5	0.4	
Liver transplants												
n	170	313	412	468	495	614	698	700	790	899	960	989
pmp	4.4	8.1	10.7	12.1	13	16	18.1	18.2	20	22.6	24.2	25
Heart transplants												
n	97	164	232	254	287	292	278	282	317	349	336	356
pmp	2.5	4.6	6	6.6	7.5	7.6	7.2	7.3	8	8.8	8.5	9
Heart-lung transplants	5	4	2	1					1	7	4	
Single-lung + double-lung transplants												
n		2	3	10	16 + 4	17 + 19	17 + 28	27 + 49	26 + 81	26+102	40 + 95	53 + 92
pmp					0.5	0.9	1.1	1.7	2.7	3.2	3.4	3.6
Pancreas transplants												
n	9	19	21	26	24	16	24	24	27	28	25	39
pmp	0.2	0.5	0.5	0.7	0.6	0.4	0.6	0.6	0.7	0.7	0.6	1

* Acquisition period: June (last year) / June (this year).

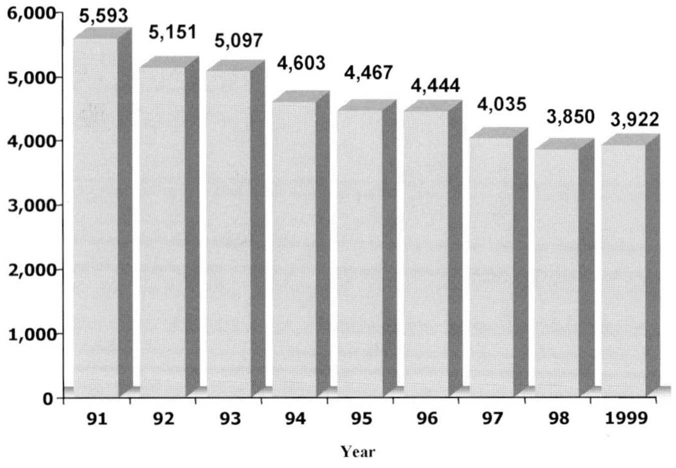

Fig. 6. Kidney waiting list evolution in Spain.

ure and criteria for admission to the waiting list has allowed a continuous decrease in the number of people waiting for a kidney until 1998, but there has been a rebound in 1999 (fig. 6).

On the other hand, the increase in the number of liver or heart transplants has not impeded a similar increase in the number of patients admitted each year to the waiting lists. The mean time to graft has been maintained (or has slightly increased) at around 2 months for heart, 3 months for a liver, and 4 months for lungs. The mortality rate for persons on the waiting list has also been maintained or slightly increased. This evolution in the outcome of the patients admitted to the waiting list each year has led to an increase in the registered number at the end of each year (table 4).

Table 4. Waiting list (WL) evolution for solid-organ transplantation in Spain

Organ	Year	Number of			WL (end of year)	Days to transplant (mean)	Mortality rate, % of overall patients
		new patients admitted	grafted patients	dead patients			
Liver	1993	640	495	31	159	72	6.2
	1996	983	700	94	297	85	7.5
	1999	1,306	960	123	403	99	7.6
Heart	1993	349	287	23	37	46	6.2
	1996	405	282	41	80	62	9.3
	1999	410	336	36	83	82	7.4
Lung	1993	34	20	0	16	43	0
	1996	103	76	8	47	148	5.6
	1999	161	135	10	47	122	4.9

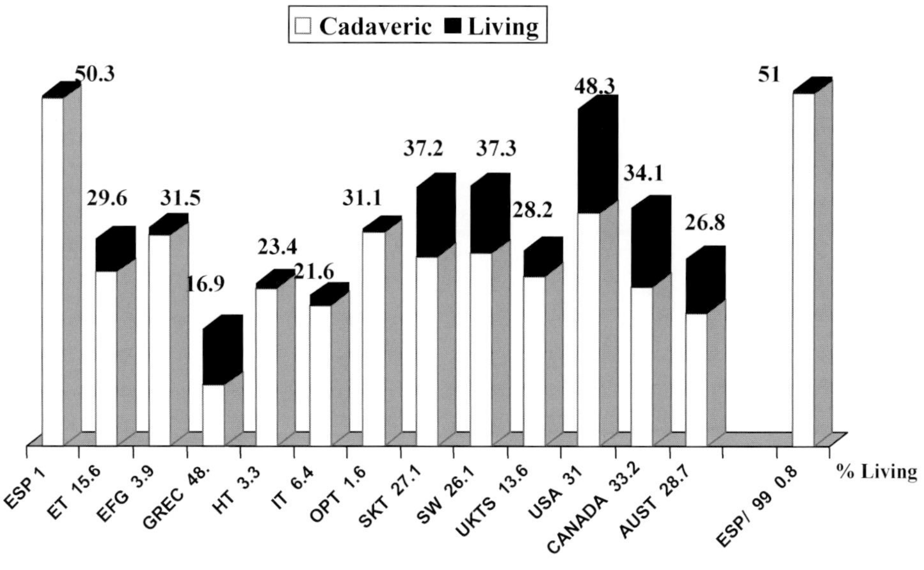

Fig. 7. Kidney transplantation from living versus cadaveric donors in different countries and regions, 1998.

Opportunities for Improvement

While waiting for possible alternatives such as artificial organs or xenografts – in order to try to face the organ shortage, there remains the only current opportunity to improve the availability of human allografts (both from living and cadaveric donors).

Living Donation Can Be a Source for Organ Transplantation
Actually, this has been the case for kidneys and tissues from the beginning of the history of transplantation procedures. Kidney transplant from living donors is highly successful not only in cases of genetic relationship between donor and recipient [11, 14]. More recently, there arose the possibility of implanting a part of a liver from a living donor, giving new opportunities for the patients, and not only for pediatric ones [15].
In Spain, kidney transplantation from living donors has been always anecdotical. This is obvious if we compare the Spanish figures with others (fig. 7). It is easy to conclude that there is an important potential source of kidneys for transplantation. Since 1995, 13 living liver transplantations have been performed, but it has to be noticed that 7 of these occurred during this year 2000, the time when also for adult recipients this procedure has been started.

Non-Heart-Beating Donors (NHBD)
These donors are also a possible source of organ for transplantation [16]. Figure 8 summarizes the number of kidneys and livers grafted in Spain during the recent years coming from NHBD. There were good results in terms of survival for both types of organs [17, 18].

Brain-Dead Donors
The process of identification, evaluation of donors and the retrieval and grafting of organs and tissues is a large and complex one, involving various steps and no fewer than 100 health care and non-health care professionals. Keeping records of all deaths in intensive care units (ICUs) and of the potential donors identified enables us

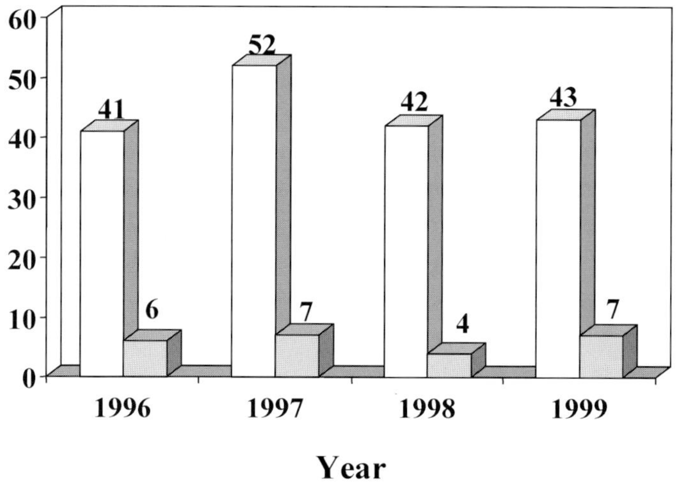

Fig. 8. Kidney (□) and liver (▒) transplants from non-heart-beating donors in Spain, 1996–1999.

to find where and when donors are lost and where and when efforts and solutions need to be implemented [9]. Published estimations of the underlying donor potential suggest that less than half of potential donors (28–60 potential donors pmp) are currently transformed into actual donors [19, 20].
Different pilot studies in this field have been started in different countries during the last years [21–27]. From these studies three main areas for improvement can be recognized: donor identification, donor management, and family approach and consent.
In 1993 this kind of data was analyzed in the Basque Country [22]. The authors concluded they were losing a potential of 17 donors pmp (8 pmp due to under-identification, 4 pmp due to family refusal, and 5 pmp due to cardiac arrest). The actual donor rate in this area at that time (1993) was 38 donors pmp. Nowadays, in 1999, the Basque Country has recorded a donor rate of 50.7 donors pmp (fig. 9).
Table 5 summarizes recent data of the continuous follow-up examinations of all ICU deaths. These follow-ups are carried out in Spain, progressively in more and more units or areas.

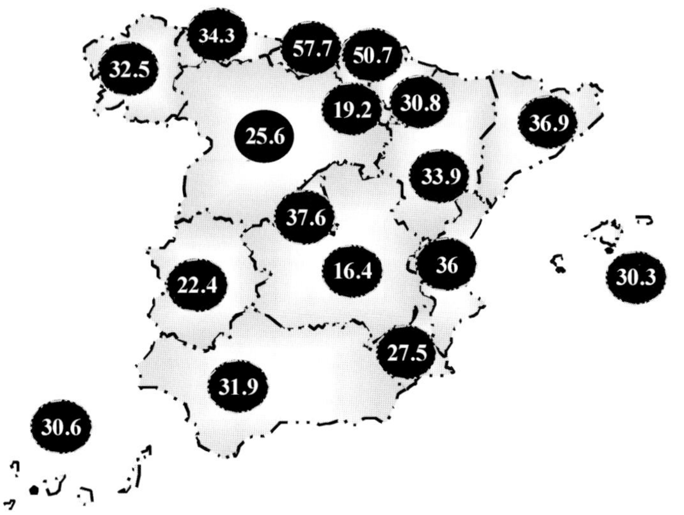

Fig. 9. Organ donation rates (ppm) in the different Spanish regions, 1999. Whole state: 33.6.

Potential donor detection is the starting point, and it is probably the most difficult step to make routine. Knowledge of the environmental characteristics – such as hospital infrastructure; mortality rates; incidence of road traffic accidents, cerebrovascular accidents, and cerebral tumors; and health resources – is mandatory. The prospective registries of brain-dead cases, complemented by retrospective medical record reviews to avoid under- or overestimation, will give us an idea about the pool of brain-dead patients and its characteristics and outcome. If this kind of study is not developed for a given area or hospital, it is possible to establish some hospital indexes that can be helpful in the estimation. A British study published in 1992 stated that 14% of all deaths in the ICU occurred in brain-dead patients [28]. The Spanish society of intensive care medicine analyzed these data over 2 years in 42 ICUs. The mean rate of deaths in the ICU occurring in brain-dead patients was 13.5%. However, when the hospital was a neurosurgery center, this rate was 20%; if no neurosurgery facilities were available, this rate was only 8% [29]. The rate of unidentified organ donors varies in the studies mentioned above between 4 and 12%. Obviously, the goal should be to identify 100% of potential donors.

During the time it takes to evaluate a donor, satisfy all legal requirements, acquire consent, and organize the logistics of retrieval, it is necessary to maintain organ viability. This period of time can be as long as 24 h, or even longer. The process is in the direct responsibility of the physician in charge at the ICU, but is also subject to surgical constraints, and time works against the entire process. In different studies [22–24], 10–14% of donors presented with hemodynamic impairment or uncontrollable sepsis, factors that contraindicate donation. In the 1997 Spanish audit, 12% of all detected potential donors presented with this problem [30]. 8% of all potential donors were lost because of irreversible cardiac arrest in the 1998 Spanish audit [27], but only 1.7% of all potential donors presented cardiac arrest during 1999 (table 5). The promotion of research and educational programs to reduce such problems should be mandatory. New techniques or therapeutic strategies that could be helpful should be widely introduced. Nevertheless, there will always be a gap that can probably only be minimized with the development of non-heart-beating donor programs.

Family refusals in Spain account for a loss of more than 350 donors, or nearly 9 donors pmp, per year. In most countries, family consent is mandatory for donation, and family refusal rates are very high [31–33]. This has led to an extended debate between authors who maintain that strict presumed consent laws are absolutely necessary and those who support the consultation of relatives [13, 34, 35]. In 1995, a Spanish survey found that most citizens (66%) are against a change in the current practice and only 6% believe that retrieval of organs should be allowed without elicitation of the family's wishes [36, 37], a practice that, as many note, could be perceived as an abuse of authority or even an insult to the family. In a more recent survey in 1999 [38], the percentage of people who would not accept such a change has decreased to 62%, and 16% think that it could be a way to improve organ availability or a sign of society's solidarity. Still 50% of the Spanish population hold the view that the family must be always approached, and just 31% think that the family should only be approached if there is no information about the deceased person's wishes. More than 95% of the general Spanish population have a favorable opinion of donors and donors' families, but the current family refusal rate is over

Table 5. Follow-up of brain death epidemiological data in the Spanish ICUs

	Year	
	1998	1999
Area	INSALUD (40%)	INSALUD + ANDALUCIA + NAVARRA (60%)
Number of hospitals	42	60
Deaths in ICU	6,230	10,616
Brain deaths (% of all ICU deaths)	783 (12.5%)	1,387 (13.1%)
Undetected	31 (4%)	23 (1.7%)
Med. contraindicated	228 (29%)	380 (27.4%)
Potential donors	524	984
No legal certification / coronar refusal	10	7
Managemant problems / cardiac arrest	43	55
Family refusals	103 (20% of 509 interviews)	227 (23.6% of 961 interviews)
Lack of adequate recipient/logistics	13	9
Actual donors	366 (67% of potential donors)	676 (68.7% of potential donors)

Table 6. Family refusals. Analysis of 361 cases in 1998

	Positive outcome	Negative outcome	p
n	287	74	
	%	%	
Male	81	77	n.s.
Female	19	23	
Age, years			
≤35	90	10	< 0.05
>35*	75–80	20–25	
Type			
Brain death	79	21	< 0.05
Non-heart-beating donor	90	10	
Judicial case	86	14	< 0.05
Non-judicial case	76	24	
Family members present in the interview			
1	95	5	< 0.05
2–5	80	20	
>5	70	30	
Family satisfaction with human treatment			
Satisfied	90	10	< 0.05
Unsatisfied	76	24	
Clear claims	54	46	
Family satisfaction with medical attention			
Satisfied	90	10	< 0.05
Unsatisfied	75	25	
Clear claims	52	48	

n. s. = Not significant.
* Variable depending on the different age groups.

21%. Thus, there is a difference between the attitude toward the hypothetical situation evaluated in general surveys and the attitude toward the real situation when a relative has died and the donor option is presented.

During 1998 a total of 361 donation processes could be analyzed, both from the perspective of the family and that of the transplant coordinator [39]. Table 6 summarizes some of the factors showing some significant relation with the positive or negative outcome. In addition, there were some other analyzed parameters that did not show any relation, such as cause of death, religion of the deceased or the family, the knowledge of somebody grafted or on the waiting list or the relationship between the decider and the deceased. From these and some other published data [27, 40–43] the investigators have identified different points that deserve special attention when approaching the grieving families:

- Proper information and treatment during all the medical processes, both from the human and medical side, are absolutely determinant.
- Specially trained staff should make the approach. Development of training programs specifically designed for this purpose, with the help of psychologists and communication experts, is deemed mandatory.
- It is necessary to make a comprehensive approach along with offers of help, not simply an interview requesting organ donation.
- The first approach should be carefully prepared, using all available information about the family members in deciding the optimum timing and place. Before starting with the interview, it is mandatory to ensure that the family members have already understood that their relative is dead; the requesting interview must be decoupled from the communication of death. Further approaching after an initially negative answer can be attempted with appropriate arguments directed toward the reversal of the refusal.
- The staff should never show that they are in a hurry.
- All interviews need to be evaluated in a follow-up by the coordinating team, so that all previous errors can be avoided. The most frequent errors are: to get angry, not to follow the rhythm of assimilation of the relatives, to interrupt the family, etc.
- The staff should never forget they are there to help and to be useful and never to disturb anyone. They should remember that most families believe that donation provides a positive outcome from death, and helps with the grieving process. It is known that 100% of donor families would donate again, and 30% of families that denied the donation would have made the opposite decision 1 year later [43–45].

References

1 Ley Española sobre extracción y trasplante de órganos. 30/1979 de 27 Octubre. BOE 6/11/79.
2 Real Decreto por el que se regulan las actividades relativas a la utilización de Tejidos Humanos, 411/1996 de 1 Marzo. BOE 23/3/96.
3 Real Decreto por el que se regulan las actividades de obtención y utilización clínica de órganos humanosy la coordinación territorial en materia de donación y trasplante de órganos y tejidos. 2070/1999, de 30 Diciembre. BOE 4/1/00.
4 Matesanz R, Miranda B, Felipe C: Organ procurement in Spain: The impact of transplant coordination. Clin Transplant 1994;8:281–291.
5 Miranda B, González-Posada JM: Principles for allocation of cadaver organs to transplant recipients and coordinating procedures in Spain; in Tourraine JL, et al. (eds): Organ Allocation. Lancaster, Kluwer, 1998, pp. 3–21.
6 Matesanz R, Viedma MA: Transplant organizations. Regional – National – International? in Matesanz R, Miranda B (eds): Organ Donation for Transplantation. Madrid, Aula Médica, 1996, Spain, pp 47–56.
7 Abbing R: Organ and tissue transplantation. A subject for European Concern. Study Report for the Council of Ministers of Health of the Member States of the European Union (1994).
8 Evans RW, Orians CE, Asher NL: The potential supply of organ donors. An assessment of the efficiency of organ procurement in the USA. JAMA 1992;267:239–246.
9 Council of Europe Transplant Newsletter, vol 4, No. 1, 1999. International figures on organ donation and transplantation. From 1998. Council of Europe. Consensus Document: Matesanz R, Miranda B (eds): Meeting the Organ Shortage. Madrid, Aula Médica, 1999.
10 Hariharan S, Johnson CP, Bresnahan BA, Taranto SE, Mcintosh MJ, Stablein D. Improved graft survival after renal transplantation in the United States, 1988 to 1996. N Engl J Med 2000;342:605–612.
11 UNOS data Registry. Disposable in URL: http://www.unos.org
12 Dew MA, Switzer GE, Goycoolea JM, Allen AS, DiMartini A, Kormos RL, Griffith BP: Does transplantation produce quality of life benefits? A quantitative analysis of the literature. Transplantation 1997;64:1261–1273.
13 First MR: Transplantation in the nineties. Transplantation 1992;53:1–11.
14 Gjertson DW, Cecka JM: Living unrelated kidney transplantation. Kidney Int 2000;58:491–499.
15 Cho YW, Terasaki P, Cecka JM: Transplantation of kidneys from donors whose hearts have stopped beating. N Engl J Med 1998;338:221–225.

16 Marcos A Right lobe living donor liver transplantation: A review. Liver Transplant 2000;6:3–20.
17 Alvarez J, Sanchez-Fructuoso A, del Barrio R, Prats MD, Torrente J, Illescas ML, Mateos P, Barrientos A: Donación de Organos en asistolia. Resultados del Hospital Clínico S. Carlos. Nefrología 1998;XVIII:47–53.
18 Mañez R, et al: Personal commun. (Hospital J. Canalejo, La Coruña. Spain).
19 Miranda B, Fernández Lucas M, Matesanz R: The potential organ donor pool: International figures. Transplant Proc 1997;29:1604–1606.
20 Mc Namara P, Beasley C: Determinants of familial consent to organ donation in the hospital setting; in Cecka, Terasak (eds): Clinical Transplant, 1997, chap. 21, pp 219–229.
21 Gortmaker SL, Beasley CL, Brigham LE, Franz HG, Garrison RN, Lucas BA, Patterson RH, Sobol AM, Grenvik NA, Evanisco MJ: Organ donor potential and performance: Size and nature of the organ donor shortfall. Crit Care Med 1996;24:432–439.
22 Aranzabal J, Texeira JB, Darpon J, et al: Capacidad generadora de órganos en la CA del País Vasco: Control de calidad. Rev Esp Trasp 1995; 4:14–18.
23 Cabrer C: Aplicación del diagrama ASME al proceso de obtención de órganos para trasplante. Tesis Doctoral, Universidad de Barcelona, 1994.
24 Navarro A: Potential donors and brain death epidemiology in the region of Madrid; in Tourain JL, et al. (eds): Organ Shortage: The Solutions. Dordrecht, Kluwer, 1995, chapt. 20.
25 Miranda B, Matesanz R: International issues in transplantation. Setting the scene and flagging the most urgent and controversial issues. Ann N Y Acad Sci 1998;862:129–143.
26 Mc Namara P, Franz H, Fowler R, Evanisko M, Beasley C. Medical record review as a measure of the effectiveness of the organ procurement. Practices in the hospital. Jt Comm J Qual Improv 1997;23:321–333.
27 Miranda B, Naya MT, Cuende N, Matesanz R: The Spanish model of organ donation. Curr Opin Organ Transplant 1999;4:109–117.
28 Gore SM, Cable DJ, Holland AJ. Organ donation from the intensive care units in England and Wales. Two year confidential Audit of deaths in Intensive Care. BMJ 1992;305:349–355.
29 Muerte encefálica y donación de órganos; in Esteban A, Escalante JL: Consejería de Sanidad y Asusntos Sociales. Madrid, 1995 (m32–581).
30 Miranda B, González-Posada JM, Sagredo E, Martín C: The potential organ donor pool. Donation process analysis. Mapfre Med 1998;9:1–8.
31 Miranda B: Aspects Juridiques et Législatifs des Transplantations d'organes: Transplantations d'Organes en Europe; Science et Conscience. European Postgraduate Training Institute of Health Care EURO COS. European Parliament. Strasbourg, France, 1994.
32 Nathen H, Jarrell B, Broznik B, et al: Estimation and characterisation of the potential organ donor pool in Pennsylvania. Transplantation 1991;51: 142–149.
33 Garrison R, Beutley F, Raque G, et al: There is an answer to the shortage of organ donors. Surg Gynecol Obstet 1991;173:391–396.
34 Roels L, Varenterghem Y, Waer M, et al: Effects of a presumed consent law on organ retrieval in Belgium. Transplant Proc 1991;23:546.
35 Matesanz R: El consentimiento informado en la donación de órganos. El Modelo Español; in Matesanz R, Miranda B (eds): Coordinación y Trasplantes. Madrid, Aula Médica, 1995, pp 143–160.
36 Martín A, et al: Donación de órganos y trasplantes. Aspectos psicosociales. Nefrología 1991; 11(suppl 1):62–68.
37 Martín A, Martínez JM, López Marinez S: Encuesta sociológica sobre la donación de órganos. El Modelo Español; in Matesanz R, Miranda B (eds): Coordinación y Trasplantes. Madrid, Aula Médica, 1995;143–160.
38 Martin A, et al: General Survey on Organ Donation in Spain. 3rd Survey corresponding to 1999 (in preparation).
39 Martin A, Martinez J, Lopez S: Analysis of 361 Family requesting processes. Int J Psychol (in press).
40 Gallup Survey: The USA public's attitudes toward organ transplantation – organ donation. Princeton, NJ, Gallup Organization, 1987.
41 Franz HG, DeJong W, Wolfe SM, Nathan H, Payne D, Reitsma W, Beasley C: Explaining brain death: A critical feature of the donation process. J Transplant Coord 1997;7:14–21.
42 Evanisko MJ, Beasley CL, Brigham LE, Capossela C, Cosgrove GR, Light J, Mellor S, Poretsky A, McNamara P: Readiness of critical care physicians and nurses to handle requests for organ donation. Am J Crit Care 1998;7:4–12.
43 De Jong W, Franz HG, Wolfe SM, Nathan H, Payne D, Reitsma W, Beasley C: Requesting organ donation: An interview study of donor and non donor families. Am J Crit Care 1998;7:13–23.
44 Gómez P, Santiago C, Moñino A, Dominguez JM: Obtención del consentimiento familiar para la donación. Relación de ayuda. Rev Esp Trasplantes 1994;3:7–14.
45 Frutos MA, Serrano B, Rando B, Ruiz P, Rosel J: Actitudes de las familias de donantes y no donantes de órganos. Rev Esp Trasplantes 1994; 3:163–169.

Chirurgische Gastroenterologie Interdisziplinär

Chir Gastroenterol 2002;18(suppl 1):18–23

Spenderorgane im Grenzbereich bei der Herz- und Lungentransplantation: Quantifizierung der Transplantatqualität, Grenzen der Akzeptanz

A. Haverich G. Warnecke S. Fischer A. Görler M. Wilhelmi M. Strüber

Klinik für Thorax-, Herz- und Gefäßchirurgie, Medizinische Hochschule Hannover

Schlüsselwörter

Herz-Lungen-Transplantation · Spenderorganmangel · Grenzwertige Spenderorgane

Key Words

Heart lung transplantation · Donor shortage · Critical donor organs

Zusammenfassung

Seit kurzem verfügbare Daten unseres thorakalen Organtransplantationsprogramms sowie der International Society for Heart and Lung Transplantation zeigen einen eindeutigen Zusammenhang zwischen Spenderorgankriterien und dem Auftreten von Komplikationen im Langzeitverlauf nach Herz- oder Lungentransplantation. So sind insbesondere Spenderalter und Ischämiezeit des Organs nicht nur mit Komplikationen in der frühpostoperativen Phase, sondern mit dem Auftreten von chronischer Organabstoßung und auch mit dem Langzeitüberleben korreliert. Hieraus muss geschlussfolgert werden, dass einer weiteren Lockerung der Spenderkriterien für Herzen und Lungen zur Transplantation, wie sie in Anbetracht des kontinuierlichen Spenderorganmangels erwogen werden, nicht zugestimmt werden kann, um nicht die Langzeitergebnisse für den einzelnen Patienten zu gefährden.

Summary

Critical Donor Organs for Heart and Lung Transplantation: Quantification of Transplant Quality, Limits of Acceptance

Recent data from our thoracic organ transplantation program as well as from the international society for heart and lung transplantation show a strong correlation between donor organ criteria and the incidence of complications during the long-term follow-up after heart or lung transplantation. Particularly impressive is the correlation of both donor age and donor organ ischemic time with the incidence of chronic rejection, i.e., transplant vasculopathy and bronchiolitis obliterans, and with long-term survival. It is concluded that donor organ criteria, with special respect to donor age and ischemic time, should not be expanded in clinical heart and lung transplantation, as is discussed in order to reduce the donor organ shortage that currently plagues clinical thoracic organ transplantation. This will avoid critically compromising long-term results for our patients.

Einleitung

Die Transplantation thorakaler Organe hat sich in den vergangenen 3 Jahrzehnten zu einem etablierten Verfahren für terminale Herzinsuffizienz und terminale Lungeninsuffizienz entwickelt. Seitens der Chirurgie sind in den letzten 15 Jahren erhebliche technische Verbesserungen erzielt worden. So sank die perioperative Letalität für die kombinierte Herz-Lungen-Transplantation von 24% im Jahr 1987 auf 14% im Jahre 1999. Besonders beeindruckend war das Absinken der operativen Sterblichkeit bei der Doppellungentransplantation von 50% im Jahr 1987 auf 16% im Jahr 1990 (Jahresstatistik der International Society for Hart and Lung Transplantation, ISHLT). Für die Herztransplantation wurden vergleichbare Daten erhoben. In den vergangenen 10 Jahren war bezüglich Operationstechniken und Verbesserung der perioperativen Ergebnisse keine wesentliche Änderung mehr zu vermerken. Verfeinerung der immunsuppressiven Therapie, Optimierung der Konservierung von Herz und Lungen sowie intensivierte Nachbeobachtungsprogramme führten zu einer weiteren Verbesserung der Patientenversorgung. Dennoch konnte im vergangenen Jahrzehnt keine Verbesserung der Prognose der Patienten erzielt werden. Dies gründete sich zum einen auf die Tatsache, dass im zunehmen-

KARGER

Fax +49 761 452 07 14
E-mail Information@Karger.de
www.karger.com

Accessible online at:
www.karger.com/journals/cga

Prof. Dr. A. Haverich
Klinik für Thorax-, Herz- und Gefäßchirurgie
Medizinische Hochschule Hannover
Carl-Neuberg-Straße 1, D-30625 Hannover (Deutschland)
Tel. +49 511 532-65 81, Fax -54 04
E-mail haverich@thg.mh-hannover.de

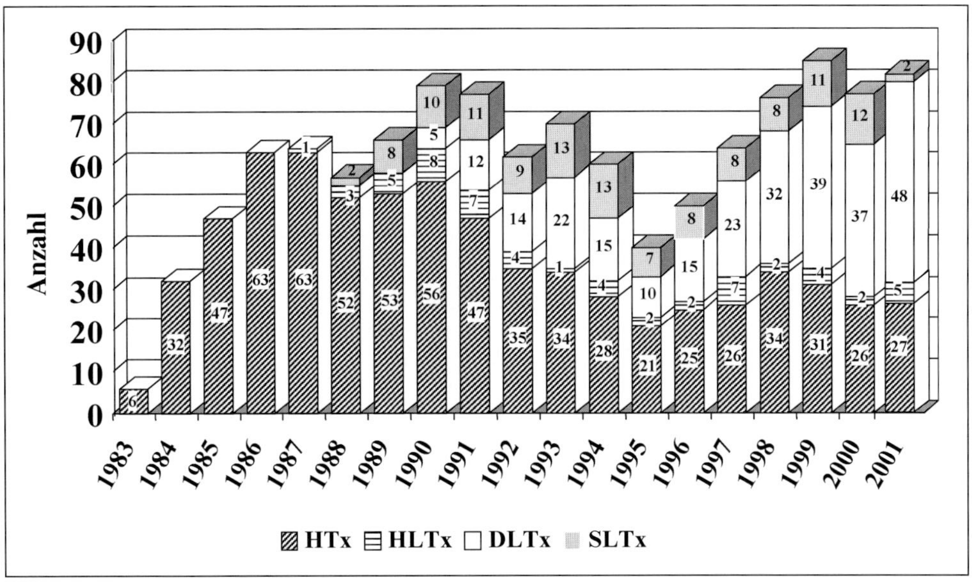

Abb. 1. Anzahl der Transplantationen pro Jahr. HTx = Herztransplantation; HLTx = Herz-Lungen-Transplantation; DLTx = Doppellungentransplantation; SLTx = Einzellungentransplantation.

den Umfang als kritisch einzuschätzende Spenderorgane verwandt wurden, zum anderen Probleme der chronischen Abstoßung bis dato nicht gelöst sind. Diese schlagen sich insbesondere auf die Langzeitprognose 5 und 10 Jahre nach Transplantation nieder und sind so bei der Herz- und der Lungentransplantation wesentlicher Faktor für das Spätversterben nach Organübertragung.

Insgesamt konnte seit 1990 weder in Deutschland noch im europäischen Bereich, noch international eine wesentliche Steigerung der thorakalen Organtransplantation erzielt werden. Dies gründete sich ausschließlich auf die mangelnde Verfügbarkeit geeigneter Spenderorgane. Dem wachsenden Druck von Seiten der Warteliste wurde durch Akzeptanz von Organen begegnet, für die noch wenige Jahre vorher klare Ausschlusskriterien für die Transplantation galten. Im Folgenden soll erörtert werden, wie sich die Spenderkriterien in den vergangenen 20 Jahren gewandelt haben und welchen Einfluss die Akzeptanz kritischer Spenderorgane auf das Transplantationsergebnis im Bereich der Herz- und Lungentransplantation nahmen. Abschließend werden Ergebnisse mit einem neuen Konservierungsverfahren vorgestellt und der Einfluss auf postoperative Lungenfunktion und Intensivaufenthalt darstellt.

Material und Methoden

In der chirurgischen Klinik der Medizinischen Hochschule Hannover wurde retrospektiv analysiert, welche Spenderkriterien, insbesondere für die Lungentransplantation, in den vergangenen 10 Jahren akzeptiert wurden, und an welchen Stellen ein Wandel eingetreten ist. Anhand der Daten der ISHLT wurde der Einfluss verschiedener Risikofaktoren für die Langzeitfunktion von Herz- und Lungenimplantaten auf Überleben und chronische Abstoßung untersucht.

Ergebnisse

Abbildung 1 zeigt die Entwicklung der Herz- und Lungentransplantation an der Medizinischen Hochschule Hannover, aufgeschlüsselt in die Jahresleistung für Herz-Lungen-, Doppellungen-, Einzellungen- und Herztransplantationen. Es wird ersichtlich, dass im Bereich der Herztransplantation und der Herz-Lungen-Transplantation keine Steigerung zu verzeichnen war, insbesondere aufgrund der mangelnden Verfügbarkeit passender Spenderherzimplantate. Die Steigerung im Bereich der Lungentransplantation (Einzel- und Doppellunge) war auf die zunehmende Akzeptanz früher als kritisch angesehener Spenderorgane zurückzuführen.

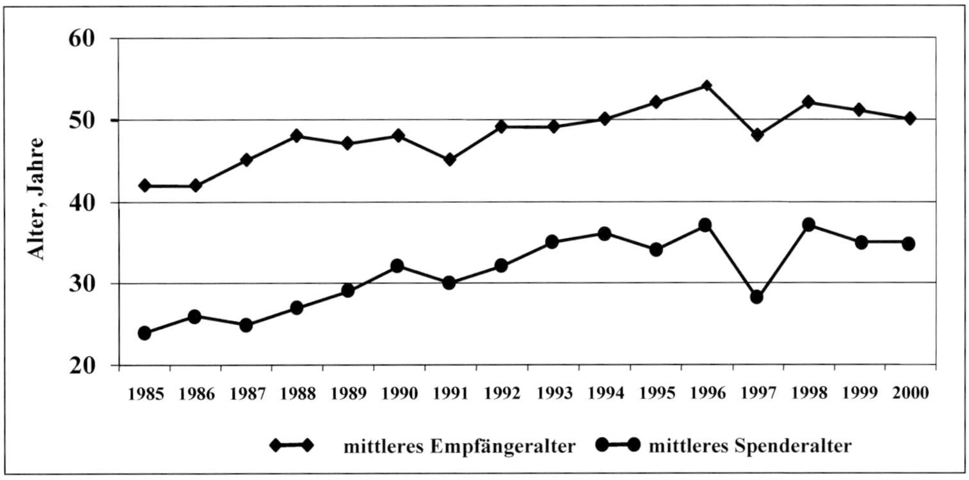

Abb. 2. Alter der Spender und Empfänger bei Herztransplantationen (Transplantatempfänger ab 18 Jahre).

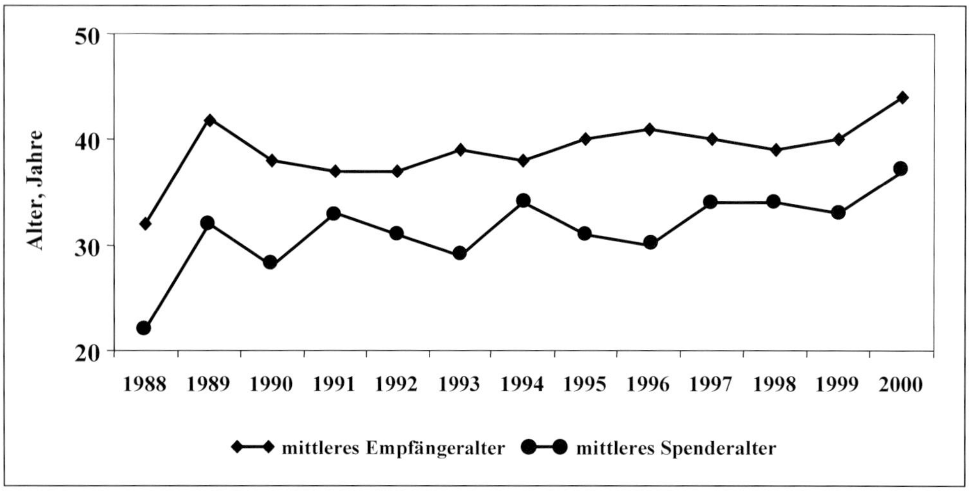

Abb. 3. Alter der Spender und Empfänger bei Lungen- und Herz-Lungen-Transplantationen (Transplantatempfänger ab 18 Jahre).

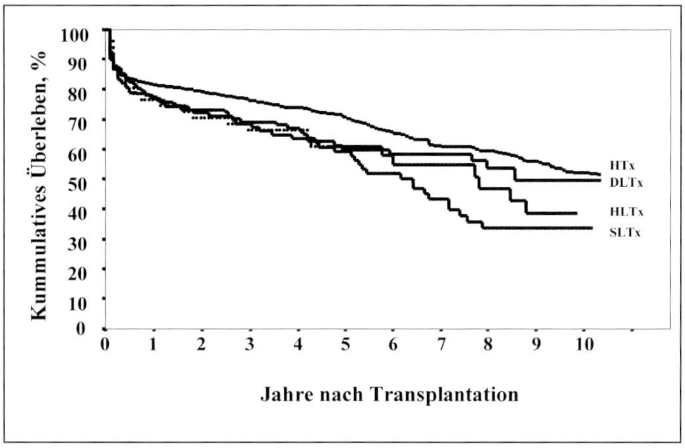

Abb. 4. Kumulatives Überleben der Patienten nach Transplantation.

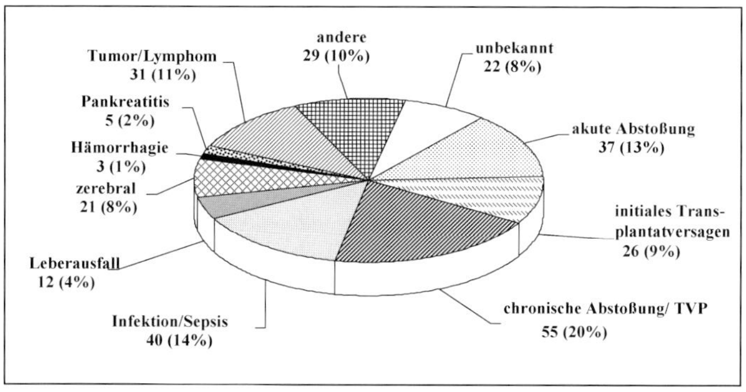

Abb. 5. Todesursachen nach Herztransplantation. GF = Transplantatversagen; TVP = Transplantatvaskulopathie.

Abbildung 2 stellt die Entwicklung für das Alter von Spender und Empfänger bei Herztransplantation in den vergangenen 15 Jahren an der Medizinischen Hochschule Hannover dar. Abbildung 3 zeigt die Veränderungen im Bereich der Lungentransplantation und in der Herz-Lungen-Transplantation. Ausgehend von einem mittleren Spenderalter von 23 Jahren im Jahre 1988 stieg danach die Altersgrenze bis auf 33 Jahre für die Lungentransplantation im Jahre 2001 an. Bei der Herztransplantation war der Anstieg von 1985 (Spenderalter 24 Jahre) bis 2001 mit 33 Jahren ebenfalls signifikant. Interessanterweise ist eine vergleichbare Zunahme des Alters auch in den Empfängeraltersklassen zu sehen, was den gestiegenen Bedarf an Transplantaten aufgrund erweiterter Spenderkriterien widerspiegelt.

In Abbildung 4 sind die langfristigen Überlebensraten bis 10 Jahre nach Herztransplantation, Doppellungen-, Herz-Lungen- und Einzellungentransplantation wiedergegeben. Es zeigt sich, dass 5 Jahre nach dem Eingriff Herztransplantate mit 70% und Einzel-, Doppel- und Herz-Lungen-Transplantate mit 60% deutlich unterschiedliche Überlebensraten widerspiegeln, wobei zwischen den einzelnen Formen der Lungentransplantation nicht unterschieden werden kann. Jenseits der 5-Jahres-Grenze sind die Zahlen für die Lungentransplantation zu gering, um statistisch signifikante Ergebnisse hervorbringen zu können. 17 Jahre nach Herztransplantation leben noch 33% der an der Medizinischen Hochschule Hannover Transplantierten. Eine Übersicht der Todesursachen nach Herztransplantation (Abb. 5) zeigt, dass ein initiales Transplantatversagen in 9% der Fälle verantwortlich ist. Die chronische Abstoßungsreaktion weist hingegen einen Anteil von 19% auf. Für die Herz-Lungen- und Lungentransplantation beträgt der Anteil an der Gesamttodesursachenstatistik für das initiale Transplantatversagen 2% und für die chronische Abstoßungsreaktion 23%. Fast die Hälfte dieser Patienten stirbt an Komplikationen, bedingt durch Infektionen und Sepsis (Abb. 6). Tabelle 1 gibt die erweiterten Indikationen für die Herztransplantation auf der Empfängerseite wieder. Die einzelnen Kriterien, wie sie 1985 für unser Herztransplantationsprogramm galten, zeigen die erhebliche Einschränkung bei der Empfängerauswahl. Im Gegensatz dazu werden nach den zur Zeit geltenden Kriterien sowohl Babys als auch Empfänger (entsprechendes biologisches Alter) bis zu 70 Jahren akzeptiert, Diabetiker nicht mehr von einer Herztransplantation ausgeschlossen, und auch die periphere arterielle Verschlusskrankheit stellt keine Kontraindikation dar. Viele der heute transplantierten Patienten haben eine koronare Bypass- oder Klappenoperation hinter sich, so dass vorangegangene herzchirurgische Eingriffe keine Kontraindikationen mehr darstellen. Auch eine Krebserkrankung in der Vorgeschichte gilt nicht als Ausschlusskriterium, wenn eine Rezidivfreiheit über einen Zeitraum von 5 Jahren vor Aufnahme auf die Warteliste nachweisbar ist. Im Jahr 1985 wurden Retrans-

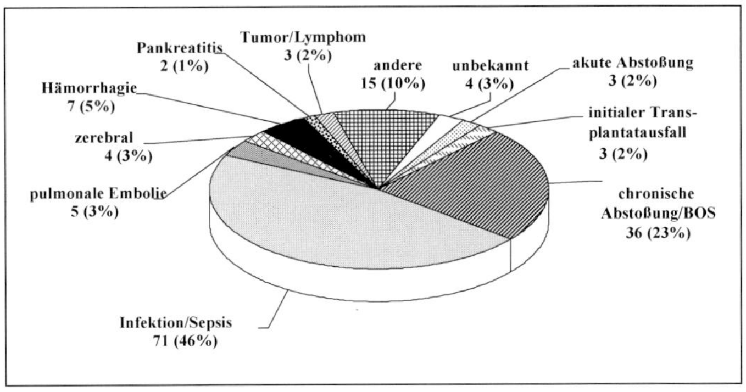

Abb. 6. Todesursachen nach Herz-Lungen- und Lungentransplantation.

Tab. 1. Erweiterte Empfängerindikationen an der Medizinischen Hochschule Hannover 1985

Alter 10–15 Jahre
Kein Diabetes mellitus
Keine periphere arterielle Verschlusskrankheit
Keine Schlaganfallanamnese
Keine Voraperation am Herzen
keine Malignomanamnese
Niedriger PVR
Keine Retransplantation

plantationen weder akut noch chronisch vorgenommen. Das hat in den vergangenen 15 Jahren eine deutliche Änderung erfahren. Zahlen mit Retransplantationen im Eurotransplant-Bereich für chronisches Transplantatversagen weisen sogar eine fast vergleichbare Überlebensrate auf wie die nach Ersttransplantation.

Ähnliche erweiterte Kriterien gelten für die Lungentransplantation, wenngleich diese aufgrund der geringen Fallzahlen nicht soweit spezifiziert sind.

In Tabelle 2 sind die Spenderkriterien für die Lungentransplantation des Jahres 1988 denen von 1998 gegenübergestellt. Anhand der Kriterien Alter, geschlechtsübergreifende Transplantation, vorangegangenes Thoraxtrauma, Oxygenierungsleistung vor Explantation, Dauer der Intubation, Größenmatch sowie projektierte Ischämiezeit wird ersichtlich, in welchem Ausmaß die Spenderkriterien

Tab. 2. Vergleich der Spenderkriterien bei Lungentransplantation

Kriterium	1988	1998
Alter, Jahre	<40	<60
Geschlecht	nein	(ja)
Thoraxtrauma	nein	ja
Oxygenierung		
(FiO_2 = 1,2), mm Hg	>500	>300
Intubationsdauer, Tage	<4	<8
Größendifferenz		
Spender/Empfänger, %	±10	±25
Ischämiezeit, h	<4	<8

für die Lungentransplantation über einen 10-Jahres-Zeitraum ausgedehnt worden sind.

Ähnliche Zahlen werden aus Statistik der ISHLT ersichtlich. Bei der Auflistung der Anzahl der Transplantate für die Lungenübertragung (aufgeschlüsselt in Einzel- und bilaterale Transplantate) zeigt sich, dass 1995 weltweit keine Steigerung der Operationsaktivität nachweisbar war. Es findet sich aber auch ein deutlicher Anstieg des mittleren Spenderalters von 24 Jahren im Jahre 1989 auf 33 Jahre im Jahre 2000 (Abb. 7).

Abbildung 8 gibt wieder, wie sich bei der Herztransplantation die 5-Jahres-Überlebensraten über einen Zeitraum von 20 Jahren entwickelt haben. Darin wird deutlich, dass zwar seit 1988 bessere Ergebnisse erzielt werden als in dem Zeitraum davor (1980–1987). Allerdings ist in den 5-Jahres-Zeiträumen danach keine wesentliche Steigerung der Überlebenszahlen mehr nachweisbar. Die Autoren stellen daher die Hypothese auf, dass die zunehmende Risikobereitschaft bei der Akzeptanz grenzwertiger Organempfänger als auch grenzwertiger Spenderorgane eine weitere Steigerung der langfristigen Ergebnisse nicht ermöglicht hat.

Abbildung 9 zeigt für die Lungentransplantation eine ähnliche Entwicklung. Unterschiede bestanden lediglich in den Vergleichszeiträumen 1997–2000 mit dem Zeitraum 1988–1992. Jenseits von 1993 konnte eine Steigerung der 5-Jahres-Ergebnisrate für die Lungentransplantation nicht erzielt werden.

Der Einfluss von Spenderalter und Ischämiezeit auf die 5-Jahres-Überlebensrate nach Lungentransplantation ist aus Tabelle 3 ersichtlich. Hieraus wird deutlich, dass ein 30-jähriger Spender auch

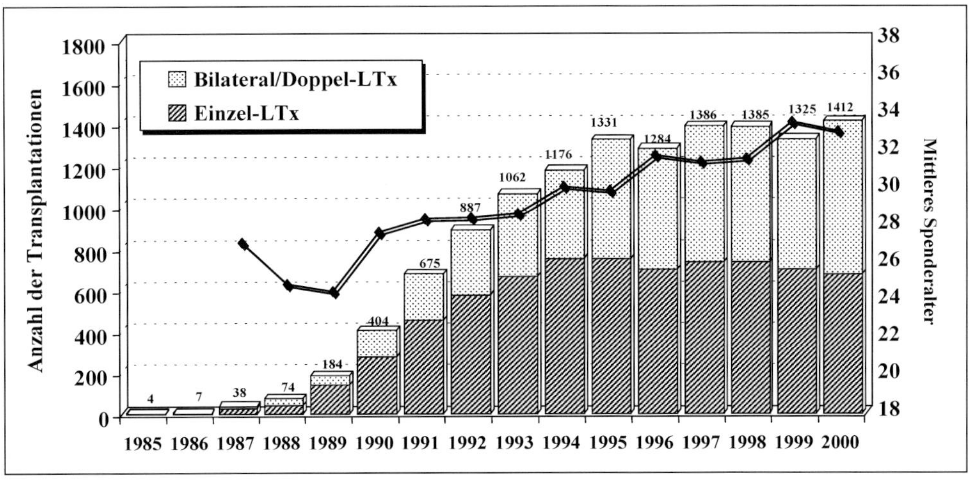

Abb. 7. Anzahl der Lungentransplantationen (LTx) weltweit zwischen 1985 und 2000 (ISHLT-Register 2000).

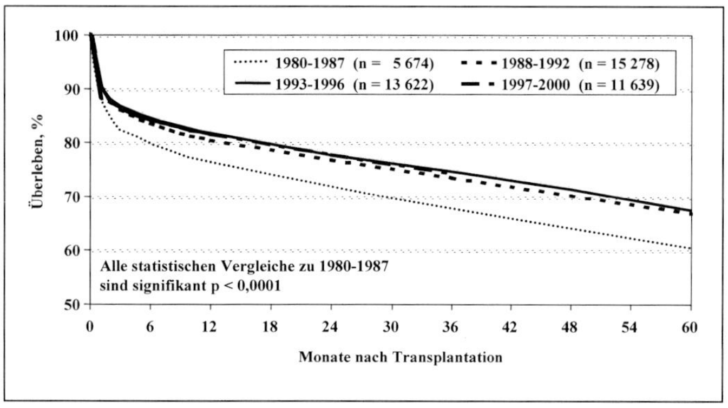

Abb. 8. Aktuarisches Überleben nach Herztransplantation (Daten der ISHLT).

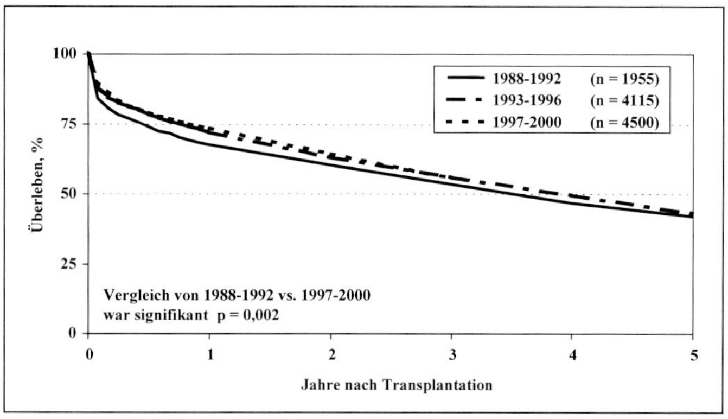

Abb. 9. Aktuarisches Überleben nach Lungentransplantation (Daten der ISHLT).

Tab. 3. Risikofaktoren für die 5-Jahres-Mortalität nach Herztransplantation (ISHLT-Registers 2000)

Variable	Odds ratio	p-Wert
Empfängeralter		
Linear		<0,0001
Quadratisch		<0,0001
Spenderalter linear		<0,0001
PVR linear		0,03
Ischämiezeit linear, h		<0,0001
0	0,61	
3	1,02	
7	2,06	
10	3,47	

mit einer Ischämiezeit von 7 h mit einer Odds ratio von 0,99 zu einem akzeptablen 5-Jahres-Überleben führt. Die Kombination aus einem älteren Spendeorgan und längerer Ischämiezeit, hier 7 h, bedingt jedoch ein 2,14-fach höheres Risiko, innerhalb von 5 Jahren nach Transplantation zu versterben.

Interessanterweise hat die Ischämiezeit auch erheblichen Einfluss auf die Bronchiolitis obliterans, die chronische Abstoßung der Lunge. Tabelle 4 zeigt, welchen Effekt eine 2- bis 8-stündige Ischämiedauer auf die Entwicklung einer chronischen Abstoßungsreaktion innerhalb eines 5-Jahres-Zeitraums nimmt.

Die Daten des ISHLT-Registers geben darüber hinaus Auskunft, welchen Einfluss die Ischämiezeit für die Herztransplantation und

Tab. 4. Risikofaktoren für Bronchitis obliterans innerhalb des 5-Jahres-Zeitraums nach Lungentransplantation (ISHLT-Register 2000)

Variable	Odds ratio	p-Wert	95%-Konfidenzintervall
Diagnose: Alpha-1-Antitrypsinmangel	0,57	0,01	0,37–0,89
Ischamiezeit linear, h			
2	0,57		
4	0,95		
6	1,16		
8	1,41		

die 1-Jahres-Mortalität hat. Eine Ischämiezeit von 0 h geht mit einer Odds ratio von 0,61 für die 1-Jahres-Mortalität einher. Die 3-stündige Ischämiezeit bedeutet eine Odds ratio von 1,02, die 7-stündige von 2,06 und eine 10-stündige Ischämiezeit vermehrt das Risiko, innerhalb eines Jahres zu versterben, um den Faktor 3,47.

Die 5-Jahres-Letalität ist linear von der Ischämiezeit des transplantierten Herzens abhängig. Nach den Daten für die Ischämiedauer ergibt sich der statistisch hochsignifikante ($p < 0,0001$) Zusammenhang zwischen Ischämiezeit und 5-Jahres-Letalität nach Herztransplantation. Diese Letalitätsrate ist ebenfalls, wie in Abbildung 10 dargestellt, eindeutig abhängig vom Alter des Empfängers und des Spenders. Interessanterweise hat auch das Spenderalter einen linearen Zusammenhang mit der chronischen Abstoßung des Herzens. Mit einem p-Wert von <0,0001 ist ein linearer Zusammenhang bei einer Gesamtzahl von 7867 Patienten (Register der ISHLT 2000) nachweisbar, wie Abbildung 11 zeigt. Hier hat das Empfängeralter bis zu 70 Jahren bezüglich der chronischen Abstoßungsreaktion oder der Transplantatvaskulopathie nach 3 Jahren keinen signifikanten Einfluss, was auch Tabelle 5 für das Spenderalter belegt (Transplantatvaskulopathie nach 5 Jahren).

Für die Lungentransplantation besteht ein eindeutiger Zusammenhang zwischen Spenderalter, Ischämiezeit und 1-Jahres-Letalität. Bei einem Empfängeralter von 20 Jahren besteht die 5-Jahres-Letalität mit einer Odds ratio von 1,16, bei einem 35-Jährigen von 0,86, bei einem 50-Jährigen von 1,14 und beim 65-Jährigen von 2,71. Diese Zahlen belegen insbesondere den außerordentlichen Einfluss des Empfängeralters für das Transplantatergebnis. Auch für die Lungentransplantation besteht für die chronische Abstoßungsreaktion zwischen Spenderalter und Auftreten einer Bron-

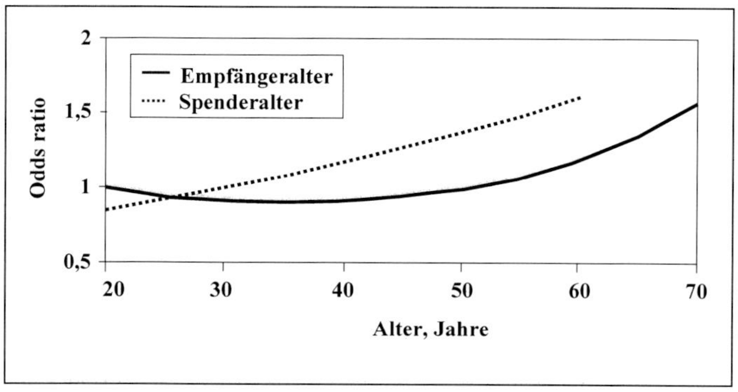

Abb. 10. Einfluss von Empfänger- und Spenderalter auf die 5-Jahres-Mortalität nach Herztransplantation (Daten der ISHLT).

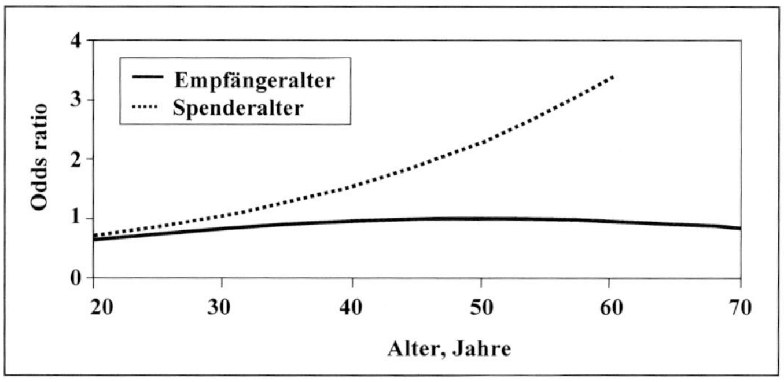

Abb. 11. Einfluss von Empfänger- und Spenderalter auf die Entstehung einer Transplantatvaskulopathie 3 Jahre nach Herztransplantation (Daten der ISHLT).

Tab. 5. Risikofaktoren für Transplantationsvaskulopathie innerhalb des 5-Jahres-Zeitraums nach Herztransplantation (ISHLT-Register 2000)

Variable	Odds ratio	p-Wert	95%-Konfidenzintervall
Diagnose:			
koronare Herzkrankheit	1,18	0,01	1,04–1,34
Empfänger weiblich	0,78	0,004	0,66–0,93
Spender weiblich	0,76	0,0002	0,66–0,88
Diagnose: kogenital	0,39	<0,0001	0,26–0,57
Spenderalter linear, Jahre		<0,0001	
20	0,74		
35	1,23		
50	2,05		
60	2,88		

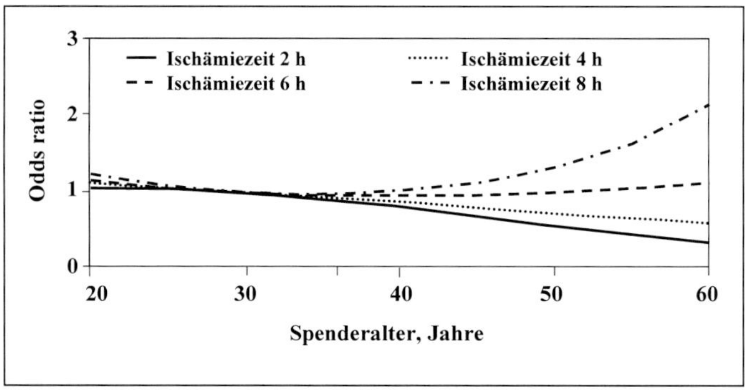

Abb. 12. Einfluss der Ischämiezeit auf die Entstehung einer Bronchiolitis obliterans 3 Jahre nach Lungentransplantation (Daten der ISHLT).

chiolitis nach 3 Jahren ein linearer Zusammenhang mit einem p-Wert von 0,009. Abbildung 12 belegt graphisch den Zusammenhang zwischen Ischämiezeit und Spenderalter bezüglich des Auftretens einer Bronchiolitis nach 3 Jahren.

Kommentar

Diese erst seit kurzem aus internationalen Statistiken und aus den eigenen Ergebnissen verfügbaren Daten belegen eindeutig, dass ein sehr enger Zusammenhang zwischen der Qualität des Spenderorgans und dem Ausgang der Transplantation besteht. Die Qualität des Spenderorgans ist in den bisher verfügbaren Untersuchungen im Wesentlichen auf das Alter und die Ischämiezeit begrenzt. Qualitative Daten wie z.B. Oxygenierung und Dauer der Intubation vor Transplantation sind nicht in ausreichender Zahl vorhanden, so dass diese Kriterien auch nicht für die Evaluation verfügbar sind.

Interessanterweise stellen sich sowohl für die Herz- als auch für die Lungentransplantation zwei Endpunkte als signifikant korreliert mit der Qualität der Spenderorgane (nach den skizzierten Kriterien evaluiert) dar. Dies sind das Überleben nach Transplantation und das Auftreten einer chronischen Abstoßungsreaktion. Hierzu ist wichtig zu wissen, dass die chronische Organabstoßung nach Herz- und Lungentransplantation den wichtigsten Risikofaktor für ein Langzeitüberleben darstellt. Damit ergibt sich ein unmittelbarer Zusammenhang zwischen der Inzidenz der chronischen Abstoßung und der Prognose für den Patienten quoad vitam. Insofern sind die Kriterien Spenderalter und Ischämiezeit nicht nur für den Endpunkt chronische Abstoßung, sondern auch für den Endpunkt Überleben des Empfängers entscheidend.

Als besonders bedeutsam wird die Ischämiezeit empfunden. Die von der ISHLT im Jahr 2000 erstmals publizierten Daten weisen den unmittelbaren Zusammenhang zwischen Ischämiezeit und chronischer Abstoßung auf. Im Zusammenhang mit derzeit diskutierten Spenderkriterien, aber auch den Allokationsregeln, muss dem *linearen* Zusammenhang zwischen Ischämiezeit und Transplantationsergebnis besondere Aufmerksamkeit geschenkt werden. Es müssen logistisch vermehrt Anstrengungen unternommen werden, um die Ischämiezeit möglichst kurz zu halten und damit der Komplikation «chronische Abstoßung» Einhalt zu gebieten.

Insgesamt weisen nationale, im Eurotransplant-Bereich gewonnene und international verfügbare Daten aus, dass der Mangel an Spenderorganen bei wachsendem Druck durch den Zustrom auf die Warteliste zu einer kontinuierlichen Aufweichung von Spenderkriterien weg von der Normalsituation in eine eben noch akzeptable Situation stattgefunden hat. Die jetzt verfügbaren Ergebnisse lassen erkennen, dass hier einer liberalen Fortsetzung dieses Trends nicht zugestimmt werden kann, da bei weiterer Ausdehnung der Kriterien, insbesondere bezüglich Spenderalter und Ischämiezeit, mit einer Verringerung der Langzeitprognose für den individuellen Patienten zu rechnen ist. Für die Transplantation der thorakalen Organe insgesamt muss ebenfalls vor einer Ausdehnung der Kriterien gewarnt werden, weil auch in größeren Kollektiven ein Absinken der 5- und 10-Jahres-Überlebensraten sowie eine deutliche Zunahme chronischer Abstoßungen zu verzeichnen sein wird. Im Gegensatz zur Transplantation von Niere und möglicherweise Leber sollten thorakale Organtransplantationsprogramme daher davon Abstand nehmen, zum jetzigen Zeitpunkt eine Erweiterung der Kriterien für die Akzeptanz thorakaler Spenderorgane vorzunehmen.

Chirurgische Gastroenterologie Interdisziplinär

Chir Gastroenterol 2002;18(suppl 1):24–28

Spenderorgane im Grenzbereich: Leber

W. O. Bechstein C. Zapletal

Chirurgische Klinik, Knappschaftskrankenhaus Bochum-Langendreer, Ruhr-Universität Bochum

Schlüsselwörter
Marginale Organe · Messung der Transplantatqualität · Verbesserung der Transplantatqualität

Zusammenfassung
Der Begriff der marginalen Organe ist in den letzten Jahren aufgrund des anhaltenden Organmangels und der wachsenden Erfahrung mit grenzwertigen Organen erheblich modifiziert worden. Spenderalter über 60 Jahre ist längst keine absolute Kontraindikation zur Organspende mehr. Vielmehr erweist sich vor allem die Leberverfettung als limitierender Faktor für eine erfolgreiche Spende. Die Marginalität der Transplantats hängt jedoch nicht allein von Spenderfaktoren ab. Auch die Entnahme selbst, die Dauer von Konservierung bzw. Ischämie/Reperfusion, die Transplantation und die Bedingungen im Empfänger können ein Spenderorgan marginal werden lassen. Messung der Transplantatqualität ist mittels klinischer und experimenteller Methoden beschrieben worden, keine hat sich jedoch als allgemein akzeptiert durchgesetzt, sodass die Erfahrung des einzelnen Operateurs noch immer eine wichtige Rolle spielt. Um zunehmend marginale Organe zur Transplantation verwenden zu können, rücken die Möglichkeiten der Transplantattherapie ins Zentrum des Interesses. Da diese oftmals experimenteller Natur sind, muss eine Überführung dieser Methoden in die Klinik vorangetrieben werden, um dem wachsenden Bedarf nach Spenderorganen zu begegnen.

Key Words
Marginal liver grafts · Quantification of graft quality · Improving graft quality

Summary
Marginal Grafts: Liver
The definition of marginal grafts has changed during recent years due to the ongoing lack of suitable organs and the growing experience with so-called marginal grafts. Donor age above 60 years is no longer a contradiction to successful liver donation, but obesity seems to be a limiting factor. Furthermore, the donation and transplantation process, conservation and ischemia-reperfusion as well as recipient-dependent factors can turn grafts into organs of marginal function. Quantification of graft quality has been evaluated by several clinical and experimental procedures, but so far none of them has become generally accepted. Experience of the transplant surgeon remains an important point in judging graft quality. To expand the donor pool possibilities of graft modifying treatment raised growing interest. Most of these therapies have not yet left the laboratory, so that it seems imminently important to bring these therapies to clinical use.

Angesichts der anhaltenden Organknappheit und wachsenden Zahl von Patienten auf der Warteliste zur Transplantation gewinnt die Frage nach der Steigerung der Organverfügbarkeit eine besondere Brisanz. Dabei ist nicht allein die absolute Zahl der Spender, sondern insbesondere die Zahl der realisierten Organentnahmen von entscheidender Bedeutung. An dieser Stelle kommt der Begriff der so genannten marginalen Organe ins Spiel.

Was sind marginale Organe?

War der Terminus «marginale Organe» ursprünglich reserviert für Organe eines älteren Spenders (>50 Jahre), bezeichnet er heute Organe, die nur eingeschränkt oder mit einem höheren Risiko zur Transplantation geeignet sind. Zur Entscheidung über die Qualität eines Spenderorgans werden verschiedene Faktoren demographi-

KARGER

Fax +49 761 452 07 14
E-mail Information@Karger.de
www.karger.com

Accessible online at:
www.karger.com/journals/cga

Prof. Dr. W. O. Bechstein
Chirurgischen Klinik, Knappschaftskrankenhaus Bochum-Langendreer
Ruhr-Universität Bochum
In der Schornau 23–25, D-44892 Bochum (Deutschland)
Tel. +49 23 42 99 32-00, Fax -09
E-mail wolf.bechstein@Ruhr-Uni-Bochum.de

scher, klinischer, laborchemischer und histologischer Art herangezogen.
Seit der Studie von Mirza et al. [1] ist bekannt, dass die Bewertung dieser Faktoren weder einheitlich noch in allen Fällen begründet ist: Dabei wurden die Spenderdaten von 30 im Zentrum Birmingham erfolgreich transplantierten Lebern, von denen 16 aus medizinischen Gründen von anderen Zentren in Großbritannien abgelehnt worden waren, mit der Frage, ob sie diese Organe akzeptieren würden, an 80 europäische Transplantationszentren geschickt. Die Rücklaufquote betrug 75%. Von den antwortenden 60 Zentren wurden 23% der Organe sofort abgelehnt und nur 37% wären von allen Zentren akzeptiert worden. Große Transplantationszentren waren dabei insgesamt weniger zurückhaltend in ihrer Akzeptanz [1].
Um die Bewertung der Spenderdaten zu vereinheitlichen und objektivierbar zu machen, wurden Bewertungsskalen entwickelt, die eine Aussage über den Erfolg der potenziell durchzuführenden Transplantation gewährleisten sollen [2]. Dabei wurden der Serumnatriumgehalt >155 mmol/l und die Gabe von Katecholamin (Dopamin >10 µg/kg Körpergewicht/min) als die wichtigsten Variablen erachtet. Auch das Alter der Spender, die Aufenthaltsdauer auf der Intensivstation, die Dauer der kalten Ischämiezeit, hypotensive Episoden und Leberwerte wurden berücksichtigt.
Der Grad der Leberverfettung, der sich in anderen Studien als relevant herausgestellt hatte, wurde nicht berücksichtigt. In einer multivariaten Analyse aus Italien, in die 311 Spenderlebern einbezogen wurden, zeigte sich eine grobtropfige Verfettung von >25% als einziger unabhängiger Risikofaktor in Bezug auf das Überleben der Empfänger. Die Rate der verspäteten Organfunktion und der primären Nichtfunktion betrug insgesamt 65%. Die feintropfige Leberverfettung blieb ohne signifikanten Einfluss [3]. Ein einfacherer Screening-Parameter zum Ausschluss einer schwerwiegenden Leberverfettung ist ein Spendergewicht von >100 kg, der in einer Studie von Mor et al. [4] mit einem erhöhten Risiko des Transplantatverlusts und einem höheren initialen Leberzellschaden vergesellschaftet war.
Ein weiterer Spenderparameter, der kontrovers diskutiert wird, ist das Spenderalter. In der internationalen Diskussion zeichnet sich ab, dass das alleinige Heranziehen des Alters keinen unabhängigen Risikofaktor für den Transplantationserfolg darstellt. Das Spenderalter beeinträchtigt nicht das Patientenüberleben, es geht jedoch mit einer erhöhten Rate an verspäteter Organfunktion, schwererem initialem hepatozellulärem Schaden und längerfristiger Cholestase einher [5].
Romero et al. [6] konnten sogar zeigen, dass auch Spenderorgane von über 80-Jährigen sicher und mit gutem Erfolg transplantiert werden können. Die Erklärung hierfür liegt in der Tatsache, dass die Leber nicht dem normalen Alterungsprozess unterworfen ist. Sie verändert sich im Hinblick auf Größe, Farbe und Konsistenz, wird dunkler und bildet eine dickere fibröse Kapsel aus [7], jedoch ist das Alter nicht automatisch mit einer Leberverfettung vergesellschaftet und normalerweise nicht in großem Ausmaß von Arteriosklerose betroffen [1].
Zusammenfassend lässt sich sagen, dass das Spenderalter allein keinen wesentlichen Einfluss auf das Organüberleben hat, dass vielmehr ausgeprägte grobtropfige Verfettung, extreme Ischämiezeiten oder beginnende Sepsis als Kontraindikationen zur Organspende gewertet werden sollten [8].
Eine einheitliche Definition über die Grenzen der Akzeptanz kann in Ermangelung eindeutig quantifizierbarer Parameter nicht gefunden werden, so dass bei aller Metaanalyse der Daten die Erfahrung des Transplanteurs von entscheidender Bedeutung bleibt [9].
Formulieren wir jedoch die eingangs gestellte Frage ein wenig anders und fragen statt «Was sind marginale Organe?» «Wodurch werden Organe marginal?», rücken andere Faktoren ins Blickfeld.

Wodurch werden Organe marginal?

Abgesehen von den Spenderfaktoren, die bereits dargelegt wurden, können zur Transplantation geeignete Organe durch den Prozess ihrer Entnahme und der Konservierung bzw. den Komplex der Reperfusion nach Ischämie, durch Empfängerkonditionen und nicht zuletzt durch eine ungünstige Kombination aller dieser Faktoren marginal werden und damit den Erfolg der Transplantation in Frage stellen (Tab. 1).
Zu den entnahmebedingten Faktoren gehören technische Probleme wie Dekapsulierung und Parenchymverletzungen der Leber, Schädigung/Verletzung des Gallengangs oder der Gefäße. Zudem verstärkt die bloße Manipulation der Leber während der Organentnahme und vor allem während der Multiorganentnahme durch die Aktivierung von Kupffer-Zellen den Reperfusionsschaden und mündet in Proteolyse, Nekrose und Verschlechterung der Mikrozirkulation [10].
Im Rahmen der Konservierung und Reperfusion nach Ischämie kann es durch unzureichendes Durchströmen mit Lösung, zu hohen Perfusionsdruck oder die Konservierungslösung selbst (die allerdings mit der UW-Lösung heute weitgehend standardisiert ist)

Tab. 1. Faktoren, die zur Marginalität von Spenderorganen beitragen

Faktor	Parameter
Spenderfaktoren	Alter, Verfettung, Länge des Aufenthalts auf Intensivstation, Hypernatriämie, Hypotension, Reanimation, Katecholamine, Infektionen
Entnahmebedingte Faktoren	Manipulation, technische Probleme, kardiozirkulatorische Instabilität des Spenders
Faktoren im Rahmen von Konservierung/Ischämie-Reperfusion	Perfusionsdruck, Konservierungslösung, Ischämiezeit, Reperfusionsschaden
Implantationsassoziierte Faktoren	Operationszeit, Transfusionen, technische Probleme
Empfängerbedingte Faktoren	präformierte Antikörper, ungenügende Leberzellmasse («small for size»), klinischer Zustand (Herz-Kreislauf-Versagen, Infektion/Sepsis)

zu einer Beeinträchtigung des Spenderorgans kommen. Schließlich stellen die Länge der Ischämiezeit und der durch die Reperfusion initiierte Schaden – der durch Sauerstoffradikale, die Aktivierung von Kupffer-Zellen und Granulozyten und die Expression von Adhäsionsmolekülen bedingt ist und in eine Beeinträchtigung der Mikrozirkulation, in Nekrose, Apoptose und hepatozellulären Schaden mündet – weitere vieldiskutierte und intensiv erforschte Themenkomplexe dar.
Hieraus ergeben sich, abgesehen von dem immer noch gültigen Gebot, die Ischämiezeit so gering wie möglich zu halten, momentan größtenteils experimentelle Ansätze für eine Verbesserung der Spenderorganqualität, mit deren Hilfe die Grenzen der Akzeptanz möglicherweise erweitert und Organspenden marginaler Spender mit größerem Erfolg realisiert werden können.
Schlechte Ausgangsbedingungen beim Empfänger müssen von Problemen, die mit der Prozedur der Implantation selbst in Zusammenhang stehen und die sich teilweise gegenseitig bedingen, unterschieden werden. Der klinische Zustand des Empfängers, die Kreislaufsituation, der Katecholaminbedarf, die Gefahr einer beginnenden Infektion oder Sepsis oder die Derangierung der Gerinnungssituation können die Operation erschweren und die Operationszeit verlängern. Eine Verlängerung der Operationszeit, Auskühlung des Empfängers und die schon präoperativ reduzierte Gerinnungsfunktion erhöhen den Bedarf intra- oder perioperativ benötigter Blutkonserven oder Gerinnungsfaktoren und wirken sich negativ auf den Transplantationserfolg aus [11, 12].
Auch die Reihenfolge der Reperfusion, ob arteriell oder portalvenös, scheint einen Einfluss auf den Transplantationserfolg zu haben. Was von Post et al. [13] experimentell untersucht und beschrieben wurde, konnte im klinischen Kontext bestätigt werden [14]. Die primäre arterielle Reperfusion unter adäquater portaler Dekompression oder die zeitgleiche arterielle und portalvenöse Reperfusion zeigt bessere Ergebnisse hinsichtlich Reperfusion und intraoperativem Verlauf.
Auch präformierte Antikörper bei Mehrfachtransplantierten oder dialysepflichtigen Patienten und ungenügende Leberzellmasse bei Splitlebertransplantation oder Lebendspenden lassen bestimmte Organe für einige Spender marginal werden.
Die Mannigfaltigkeit der Faktoren, die das Transplantationsergebnis negativ beeinflussen und deshalb marginale Bedingungen schaffen, legt die Schlussfolgerung nahe, dass nicht durch einen Faktor allein, sondern durch die Kombination verschiedener Risikofaktoren das Ergebnis negativ beeinflusst wird.

Welches Organ ist für welchen Spender marginal?

Die Kombination aus einer Hochrisikokonstellation auf Seiten des Empfängers und gleichzeitig des Spenderorgans sollte aus den genannten Gründen vermieden werden. Das bedeutet, dass ein für einen klinisch instabilen oder älteren Empfänger möglichst optimale Bedingungen bezüglich Spenderorgan, Ischämiezeit und Implantation ausgewählt werden sollten.
Ein marginales Organ, z.B. bei beginnender Leberverfettung, sollte besonders sorgfältig konserviert werden und lediglich einer kurzen Ischämiezeit ausgesetzt sein. Diese Organe können mit größerem Erfolg in klinisch stabile Empfänger implantiert werden. Marginale Organe eignen sich nicht für Lebersplitting oder «reduced size»-Transplantationen. Schwierige technische Bedingungen wie arterielle Doppelversorgung oder Größendiskrepanzen zwischen Spender und Empfänger sollten für weniger ideale Empfänger ebenfalls vermieden werden, da sie zusätzlich den Einsatz von Hochrisikotransplantaten erschweren.
Nach den Überlegungen, welche Faktoren zur Grenzwertigkeit von Spenderlebern beitragen, stellt sich die Frage, ob und welche Parameter es gibt, um die Transplantatqualität objektiv zu quantifizieren.

Quantifizierung der Transplantatqualität

Wie bereits beschrieben, haben retrospektive Analysen der Spenderdaten anhand des Transplantaterfolgs keinen eindeutigen Aufschluss über Parameter der zu erwartenden Transplantatqualität erbracht [2].
Der Grad der Verfettung gilt als einer der wichtigsten Risikofaktoren der Einschränkung der Organqualität eines Lebertransplantats. Er kann durch das Spendergewicht mit >100 kg [4] primär geschätzt werden. Zur genaueren Analyse ist die Verfettung einer histologischen Schnellschnittdiagnostik zugänglich, die jedoch in nächtlichen Zeiten der Organentnahme und -transplantation bzw. an Wochenenden und Feiertagen nicht überall zur Verfügung steht.
Ein weiterer Parameter zur Einschätzung einer verfetteten Spenderleber ist die Analyse von Aminosäuren im Effluat. Von Frankenberg et al. [15] konnten im Tierexperiment nicht nur eine vermehrte Ausschwemmung von Aminosäuren im Effluat feststellen, sondern es gelang, Grenzwerte zu definieren, die mit dem Maximum der Transaminasenausschüttung nach Lebertransplantation korrelierten. Demzufolge darf die Summe der Aminosäuren Alanin, Histidin, Valin und Leucin nicht mehr als 25 nmol/l betragen. Eine klinische Validierung dieser Studie steht noch aus. Ein weiterer Ansatz zur Analyse verfetteter Spenderlebern besteht in der Durchführung von Analysen der Gallenflüssigkeit der Spender durch Protonen-Magnetresonanztomographie. Bei signifikanter Verfettung zeigt diese ein höheres Signal von Phosphatidylcholingruppen und eine verminderte Clearance der UW-Lösung [16].
Neben all diesen Ansätzen zur Analyse der Transplantatqualität bleibt die primäre Einschätzung des erfahrenen Operateurs von Bedeutung. Der erste Blick auf das Organ, die Beschaffenheit der Ränder, die Farbe und Konsistenz des Organs sowie die Homogenität der Perfusion erlauben wertvolle Rückschlüsse auf die Qualität und können im Zweifel den Ausschlag zu weiteren Untersuchungen der Transplantatfunktion geben [9].
Ein konsequentes perioperatives Monitoring der Lebermikrozirkulation, wie sie in Heidelberg mittels Thermodiffusion routinemäßig praktiziert wird [17], erlaubt zwar keine Einschätzung des Spenderorgans vor Transplantation, jedoch eine valide Quantifizie-

rung einer Mikrozirkulationsstörung und damit des Reperfusionsschadens nach Ischämie 1 h nach Reperfusion sowie im frühpostoperativen Verlauf. Dies ermöglicht auch ein frühes therapeutisches Eingreifen mit dem Ziel einer Verbesserung der Transplantatfunktion.

Nach der Definition des Begriffs marginaler Organe, die in den letzten Jahren eine erhebliche Korrektur erfahren hat, und den Vorschlägen zur Quantifizierung der Transplantatqualität muss nun Stellung zu der Frage nach den Grenzen der Akzeptanz bezogen werden.

Grenzen der Akzeptanz

Ziel der Spenderakzeptanz eines Transplantationszentrums muss es sein, die Anzahl der Patienten auf der Warteliste mit der Zahl der zur Transplantation zur Verfügung stehenden Organe möglichst in Einklang zu bringen. Das Risiko des Versterbens auf der Warteliste sollte minimiert werden, ohne das Ergebnis nach Transplantation und insbesondere das Überleben der Patienten durch Akzeptanz von Organen oder Bedingungen «jenseits der Grenze» zu verschlechtern. Dabei müssen unter Umständen eine höhere Inzidenz von verzögerter Organfunktion oder primärer Nichtfunktion und konsekutiv eine größere Zahl von Retransplantationen in Kauf genommen werden [18].

Im Hinblick auf die Akzeptanz marginaler Organe werden zukünftig die Möglichkeiten der Transplantattherapie an Bedeutung gewinnen. Hierbei stehen experimentelle Ansätze wie die Gentherapie des Transplantats sowie Spender- und Empfängerkonditionierung zur Verfügung.

Gentherapeutisch war es im Tierexperiment durch adenovirale Vektoren möglich, den Ischämie-/Reperfusionsschaden nach Transplantation durch Reduktion der Sauerstoffradikale mittels Superoxiddismutasegen [19] bzw. die auftretende Apoptose mittels Einschleusung des *bcl2*-Gens [20] zu beeinflussen. Diese Ansätze müssen mangels geeigneter viraler Vektoren für humane Organspender und angesichts einer Vorbehandlungszeit von mindestens 48 h derzeit noch als klinisch nicht durchführbar eingestuft werden.

Unter Spender- und Empfängerkonditionierung ist die vorbereitende Therapie von Spender bzw. Empfänger auf einen bevorstehenden Stress zu verstehen. Das Prinzip besteht in der Applikation eines geringfügigen Stresses, der über die Aktivierung endogener Schutzmechanismen protektiv gegenüber dem nachfolgenden Stress wirkt. Am verbreitetsten ist das Prinzip der ischämischen Präkonditionierung, bei der durch eine kurzfristige Reperfusion nach Ischämie ein früher sofortiger und ein späterer protektiver Effekt nach darauffolgender längerer Reperfusionszeit beschrieben werden.

Dieses Prinzip wird bereits im Zusammenhang von warmer Reperfusion nach Ischämie bei großen Leberresektionen klinisch eingesetzt [21]. Experimentell zeichnen sich Erfolge der ischämischen Präkonditionierung nach Lebertransplantation [22, 23] und nach Ischämie/Reperfusion verfetteter Lebern [24] ab.

Weitere Möglichkeiten der Therapie bestehen in Modifikation der Konservierung, z. B. durch die Applikation von Sauerstoff während der Kaltlagerung [25] oder durch kontinuierliche Perfusion mit Konservierungslösung.

Ein weiterer wichtiger Interventionszeitpunkt ist die Reperfusion. Der sich zu diesem Zeitpunkt manifestierende Reperfusionsschaden konnte im Tierexperiment durch Applikation von Antioxidanzien [26, 27], Antikörpern gegen Adhäsionsmoleküle [28] oder durch pharmakologische Blockade von Kupffer-Zellen [29], durch Verbesserung der Rheologie und Bereitstellung von Sauerstoff [30] wirksam abgefangen werden. Momentan gibt es Bestrebungen, die zahlreichen experimentellen Erkenntnisse in Form von randomisierten Multicenter-Studien in die Klinik zu überführen.

Die Transplantattherapie endet jedoch nicht mit der Reperfusion im Empfänger. Auch in der frühen postoperativen Phase kann bei verzögerter Transplantatfunktion therapeutisch eingegriffen werden. Die Applikation von Prostaglandinen verbessert auch zu diesem Zeitpunkt die Transplantatfunktion [31].

Zusammenfassend ist festzustellen, dass die Kategorisierung der Transplantate als «marginale Organe», also unter erhöhtem Risiko verwendbare Organe, nicht nur vom Spender allein, sondern von allen Variablen der Transplantation abhängig ist und sich auch nur aus der Kombination dieser Faktoren ergibt. Mit den Fortschritten der Transplantattherapie können zunehmend potenzielle Spenden realisiert und das begrenzte Spenderaufkommen für den übersteigenden Bedarf besser genutzt werden. Insbesondere müssen Bestrebungen unternommen werden, die Erkenntnisse der experimentellen Forschung zeitnah der Klinik zuzuführen.

Literatur

1 Mirza DF, Gunson BK, Da Silva RF, Mayer Ad, Buckels JA, Mc Master P: Policies in Europe on 'marginal quality' donor livers. Lancet 1994;344: 1480–1483.

2 Brinceno J, Solorzano G, Pera C: A proposal for scoring marginal liver grafts. Transpl Int 2000; 13(suppl 1):S249–252.

3 Zamboni F, Franchello A, David E, Rocca G, Ricchiuti A, Lavezzo B, Rizzetto M, Salizzoni M: Effect of macrovescicular steatosis and other donor and recipient characteristics on the outcome of liver transplantation. Clin Transplant 2001;15:53–57.

4 Mor E, Klintmalm GB, Gonwa TA, Solomon H, Holman MJ, Gibbs JF, Watemberg I, Goldstein RM, Husberg BS: The use of marginal donors for liver transplantation: A retrospective study of 365 liver donors. Transplantation 1992;53:383–386.

5 Yersiz H, Shaked A, Olthoff K, Imagawa D, Shackleton C, Martin P, Busuttil RW: Correlation between donor age and the pattern of liver graft recovery after transplantation. Transplantation 1995;60:790–794.

6 Jimenez Romero C, Moreno GE, Colina RF, Palma CF, Loinaz SC, Rodriguez GF, Gonzalez PI, Garcia GI, Rodriguez RD, Moreno SC: Use of octogenarian livers safely expands the donor pool. Transplantation 1999;68:469–471.

7 Wall W: Age and liver donation. Liver Transpl Surg 1995;1:341–343.

8 Loinaz C, Gonzalez EM: Marginal donors in liver transplantation. Hepatogastroenterology 2000; 47:256–263.

9 Zamir GA, Markmann JF, Abrams J, Macatee MR, Nunes FA, Shaked A, Olthoff KM: The fate of liver grafts declined for subjective reasons and

transplanted out of a local organ procurement organization. Transplantation 2000;70:1149–1154.

10 Schemmer P, Schoonhoven R, Swenverg JA, Bunzendahl H, Thurman RG: Gentle in situ liver manipulation during organ harvest decreases survival after rat liver transplantation: Role of Kupffer cells. Transplantation 1998:27;65:1015–1020.

11 Müller AR, Platz KP, Krause P, Kahl A, Rayes N, Glanemann M, Lang M, Wex C, Bechstein WO, Neuhaus P: Perioperative factors influencing patient outcome after liver transplantation. Transpl Int 2000;13(suppl 1):S158–161.

12 Cacciarelli TV, Keefe EB, Moore DH, Burns W, Busque S, Concepcion W, So SK, Esquivel CO: Effect of intraoperative blood transfusion on patient outcome in hepatic transplantation. Arch Surg 1999;134:25–29.

13 Post S, Menger MD, Rentsch M, Gonzalez AP, Herfarth C, Messmer K: The impact of arterialization on hepatic microcirculation and leucocyte accumulation after liver transplantation in the rat. Transplantation 1992;54:789–794.

14 Noun R, Sauvanet A, Belghiti J: Appraisal of the order of revascularization in human liver grafting: A controlled study. J Am Coll Surg 1997; 185:70–73.

15 von Frankenberg M, Stachlewitz RF, Froman DT, Frey W, Bunzendahl H, Lemasters JJ, Thurman RG: Amino acids in rinse effluents as a predictor of graft function after transplantation of fatty livers in rats. Transpl Int 1999;12:168–175.

16 Melendez HV, Ahmadi D, Parkes HG, Rela M, Murphy G, Heaton N: Proton nuclear magnetic resonance analysis of hepatic bile from donors and recipients in human liver transplantation. Transplantation 2001;72:855–890.

17 Klar E, Kraus T, Bleyl J, Newman WH, Bowman HF, Hofmann WJ, Kummer R, Bredt M, Herfarth C: Thermodiffusion for continuous quantification of hepatic microcirculation – validation and potential in liver transplantation. Microvasc Res 1999;58:156–166.

18 Melendez HV, Heaton ND: Understanding 'marginal' liver grafts. Transplantation 1999;68:469–471.

19 Lehmann, TG, Wheeler MD, Schwabe RF, Connor HD, Schoonhoven R, Bunzendahl H, Brenner DA, Jude Samulski R, Zhong Z, Thurman RG: Gene delivery of CU/Zn-superoxide dismutase improves graft function after transplantation of fatty livers in the rat. Hepatology 2000;32: 1255–1264.

20 Bilbao G, Contreras JL, Gomez-Navarro J, Eckhoff DE, Mikheeva G, Krasnykh V, Hynes T, Thomas FT, Thomas JM, Curiel DT: Genetic modification of liver grafts with an adenoviral vector encoding the Bcl-2 gene improves organ preservation. Transplantation 1999;67:775–783.

21 Clavien PA, Yadav S, Sindram D, Bentley RC: Protective effects of ischemic preconditioning for liver resection performed under inflow conditions in humans. Ann Surg 2000;232:155–162.

22 Yin DP, Sankary HN, Chong AS, Ma LL, Shen J, Foster P, Williams JW: Protective effect of ischemic preconditioning on liver preservation-reperfusion injury in rats. Transplantation 1998; 66:152–157.

23 Arai M, Thurman RG, Lemasters JJ: Ischemic preconditioning of rat livers against cold storage-reperfusion injury: Role of nonparenchymal cells and the phenomenon of heterologous preconditioning. Liver Transpl 2001;7:292–299.

24 Selzner M, Calvien PA: Fatty livers in liver transplantation and surgery. Sem Liver Dis 2001; 21:105–113.

25 Minor T, Saas S, Kotting M, Nagelschmidt M, Paul A: Endischemic oxygen persufflation to improve viability of marginally preserved donor livers. Transpl Int 1998;11(suppl 1):S400–403.

26 Thies JC, Koeppel TA, Lehmann T, Schemmer P, Otto G, Post S: Efficacy of N-acethylcysteine as a hepatoprotective agent in liver transplantation: An experimental study. Transpl Proc 1997; 29:1326–1327.

27 Koeppel TA, Trauner M, Mennone A, Arrese M, Rios-Velez L, Boyer JL: Role of gluthathione in hepatic bile formation during reperfusion after cold ischemia of the rat liver. J Hepatol 1998;28:812–819.

28 Nishimura Y, Takei Y, Kawano S, Goto M, Nagano K, Tsuji S, Nagai H, Ohmae A, Fusamoto H, Kamada T: The F(ab′)2 fragment of an anti-ICAM-1 monoclonoal antibody attenuates liver injury after orthotopic liver transplantation. Transplantation 1996; 61:99–104.

29 v Frankenberg M, Golling M, Mehrabi A, Nentwich H, Thies J, Schaeffer F, Jahnke C, Bud O, Gebhard MM, Otto G, Thurman RG, Herfarth C, Klar E: Destruction of Kupffer's cells increases total liver blood flow and decreases ischemia reperfusion injury in pigs. Transplant Proc 1999; 31:3253–3254.

30 Zapletal C, Bode A, Papapostolou G, Gebhard MM, Herfarth Ch, Klar E: Hämodilution mit bovinem Hämoglobin (HBOC) vermindert den Ischämie/Reperfusionsschaden nach partiell warmer Leberischämie an der Ratte. Langenbecks Arch Surg Chir Forumband 2001;30:241–243.

31 Neumann UP, Kaisers U, Langrehr JM, Glanemann M, Müller AR, Lang M, Jörres A, Settmacher U, Bechstein WO, Neuhaus P: Administration of prostacyclin after liver transplantation. A placebo controlled randomized trial. Transplant 2000;14:70–74.

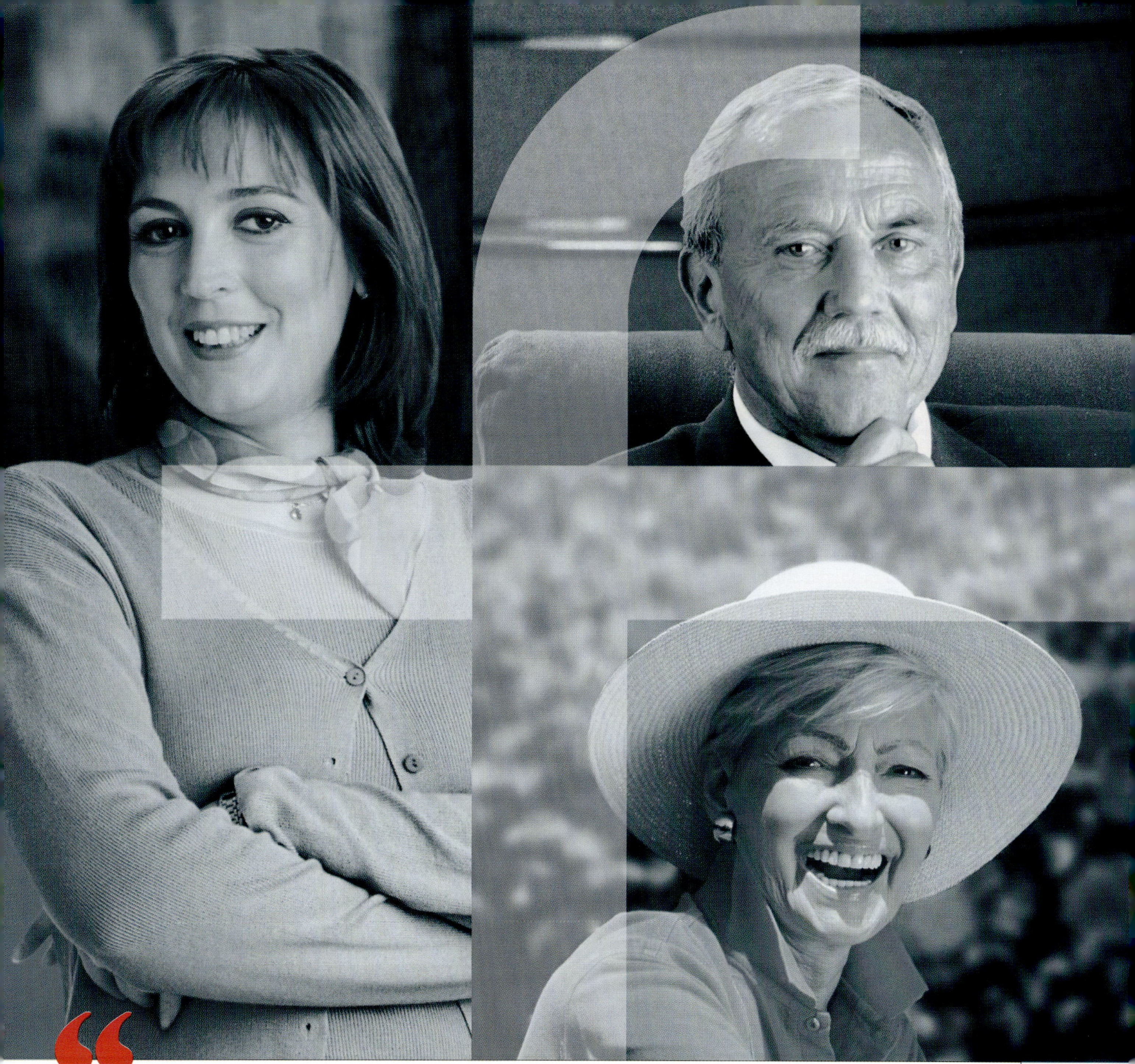

Chirurgische Gastroenterologie Interdisziplinär

Chir Gastroenterol 2002;18(suppl 1):30–33

Steigerung der Organverfügbarkeit durch Leberlebendspende

S. Nadalin M. Malagó C. E. Broelsch

Klinik für Allgemein- und Transplantationschirurgie, Universitätsklinikum Essen

Schlüsselwörter

Lebertransplantation · Leberlebendspende · Split-Lebertransplantation

Key Words

Liver transplantation · Living donor liver donation · Split liver transplantation

Zusammenfassung

Die Entwicklung der allogenen Leichenorgan-Lebertransplantation (LTx) lässt einen dramatischen Verlauf innerhalb der letzten Jahre erkennen. Während die Anzahl der durchgeführten LTx seit 1997 stagniert, steigt die Zahl neu angemeldeter Patienten auf der Warteliste kontinuierlich an. Dies führt zu zunehmenden Wartezeiten auf der LTx-Liste mit der Konsequenz, dass Patienten aufgrund der Verschlechterung ihres Zustands nicht mehr transplantierbar sind oder sogar auf der Warteliste versterben. Um den Pool der zur Verfügung stehenden Organe für die Patienten zu vergrößern und ihnen so rechtzeitig die Transplantation zu ermöglichen, wurden in den letzten Jahren neue Techniken etabliert, wie z. B. die Teilleberspende (Split-LTx) und die Lebendspender-LTx (living donor liver transplantation, LDLTx). Die LDLTx hat den entscheidenden Vorteil der Verkürzung der Wartezeit, der Planung des Eingriffs und der Verfügbarkeit eines primär gut funktionierenden Organs. Mit den zur Verfügung stehenden Methoden der Elterntransplantation oder der Leichenteil-LTx ist die Mortalität von Kindern auf der Warteliste für LTx praktisch null. Seit 5 Jahren wird als eine wesentliche Ergänzung zur Kinder-LDLTx die Erwachsenen-LDLTx durchgeführt, wobei das Risiko des Spenders dominant im Vordergrund der Erwägung und der Selektion steht. Die derzeitigen Ergebnisse von Patienten- und Transplantatüberleben nach LDLTx sind vergleichbar mit denen bei konventioneller LTx und günstiger als bei der Split-LTx. Neben der Erweiterung des Organpools bietet die LDLTx darüber hinaus die Möglichkeit, einem erweiterten Patientenkollektiv die potenziell kurative Therapie anbieten zu können.

Summary

Increase of Organ Disposability through Living Donor Liver Donation

During the last 5 years a dramatic course of cadaveric liver transplantation (LTx) was observed: While the total amount of LTxs has reached a steady state, the number of patients registered on the waiting list has been still increasing. Consequently, their general condition deteriorated during the waiting time, they were no more transplantable or even died while on the waiting list. To increase the organ disposability, new techniques have been developed: the split LTx and the living donor LTx (LDLTx). The LDLTx offers the following main advantages: shortening the waiting time, planning the operation, and optimal quality of the graft. As a result of split LTx and LDLTx the mortality of children on the waiting list was completely annulled. Since 5 years LDLTx has also been performed in adults. In this case the donor's risk and selection play a central role. The actual results of patients' and graft survival after LDLTx are comparable with those of cadaveric LTx and are better than those of split LTx. In addition to an expansion of the organ pool, LDLTx offers the possibility to extend the LTx indications.

KARGER

Fax +49 761 452 07 14
E-mail Information@Karger.de
www.karger.com

Accessible online at:
www.karger.com/journals/cga

Prof. Dr. C. E. Broelsch
Klinik für Allgemein- und Transplantationschirurgie
Universitätsklinikum Essen
Hufelandstraße 55, D-45122 Essen (Deutschland)
Tel. +49 20 17 23-1 00, Fax -59 46
E-mail Christoph.broelsch@uni-essen.de

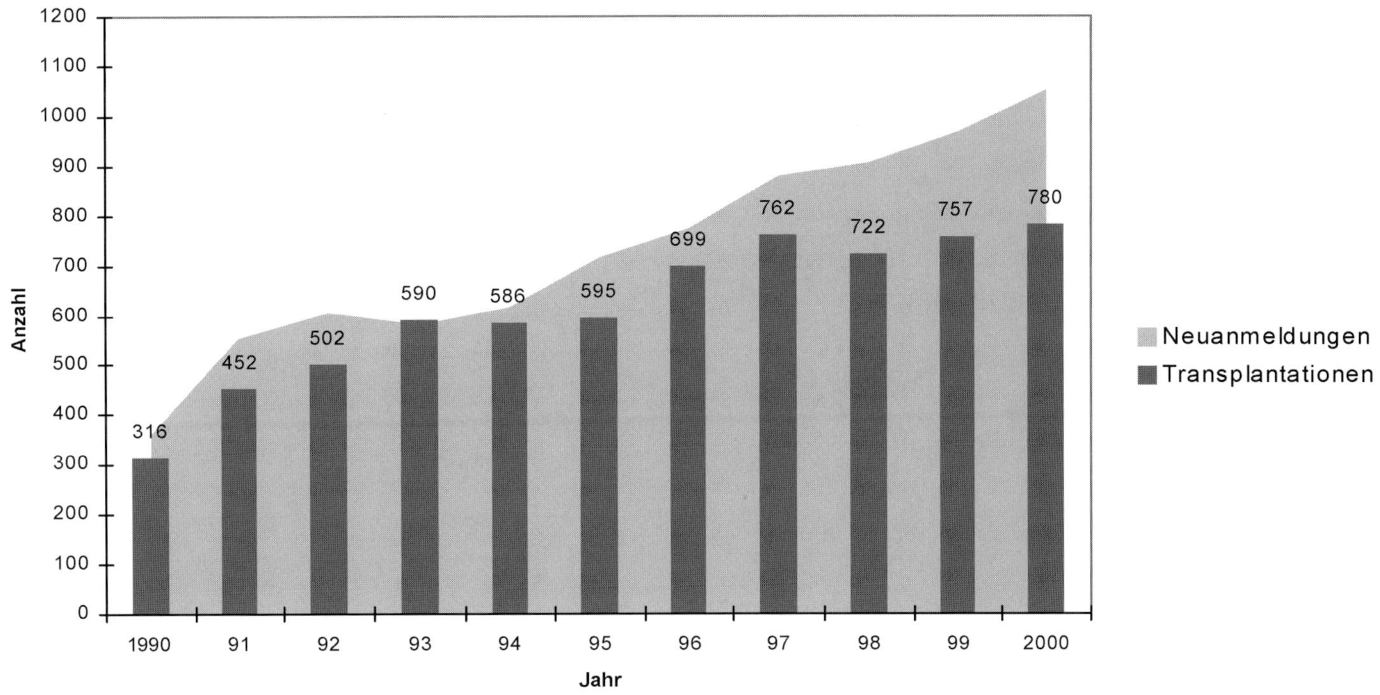

Abb. 1. Zeitverlauf der Neuanmeldungen und LTx in Deutschland [aus 1].

Die Entwicklung für die allogene Leichenorgan-Lebertransplantation (LTx) innerhalb der letzten Jahre lässt einen dramatischen Verlauf erkennen. Während die Anzahl der durchgeführten LTx seit 1997 stagniert, steigt die Zahl neu angemeldeter Patienten auf der Warteliste kontinuierlich an. Im gesamten Bundesgebiet wurden im Jahr 2000 durch postmortale Spende 589 Lebern zur Transplantation zur Verfügung gestellt. Gegenüber 1991 ist dies ein Zuwachs von 47%. Im gleichen Zeitraum verdreifachte sich jedoch die Zahl der jährlichen Neuanmeldungen zur LTx (Abb. 1). Dies führte zu steigenden Wartezeiten auf der LTx-Liste, letztendlich mit der Konsequenz, dass Patienten aufgrund der Verschlechterung ihres Zustands nicht mehr transplantierbar sind oder sogar auf der Warteliste versterben. Diese Sterberate lag 1999 bei 15% der Patienten auf der Warteliste zur LTx und etwa 8% wurden als «nicht transplantabel» gemeldet. Eine weitere Folge der langen Wartezeiten ist der steigende Anteil an schwerstkranken Patienten zum Zeitpunkt der LTx. In dieser Patientengruppe lässt sich eine deutlich erhöhte Morbidität und Mortalität nachweisen. Die ständige Erweiterung von Indikationen für eine LTx führt dabei zu einer weiteren Verschärfung der Organknappheit.

Das Haupthindernis für die Durchführung von LTx besteht meistens nicht in deren technischer Realisierbarkeit, der chirurgischen Mortalität oder der Abstoßungsproblematik, sondern in der begrenzten Anzahl von Spenderorganen im Verhältnis zur Anzahl der Patienten, denen durch eine Transplantation geholfen werden könnte. Insgesamt ist die Einstellung zur Organspende in der Bevölkerung zwar positiv, aber vergleichsweise wenige Menschen halten ihre Entscheidung schriftlich fest oder teilen diese ihren Angehörigen mit. Hier spielen verschiedene Aspekte wie eine Tabuisierung des Themas Tod oder auch die Angst, als eingetragener Spender im Fall einer intensivmedizinischen Behandlung nur im Dienste der Organspende behandelt zu werden, eine Rolle. So sind viele Angehörige, die im Krankenhaus um eine Einwilligung zur Organspende des Verstorbenen gebeten werden, unsicher, mit welcher Entscheidung sie dessen Willen wirklich entsprechen. Das deutsche Transplantationsgesetz (TPG) fordert diese Zustimmung am Totenbett, wobei in der Realität vorwiegend vom Widerspruch Gebrauch gemacht wird. Das Totensorgerecht steht über dem Lebensrecht des sterbenden Leber-, Herz- oder Lungenpatienten (§4 des deutschen TPG über die Spende, Entnahme und Übertragung von Organen, Deutscher Bundestag, 5. November 1997).

In Deutschland wurden 1999 insgesamt 1 039 Organspenden realisiert [1]. Das entspricht einer Organspenderate von 12,7 Spenden pro Million Einwohner (pmp)/Jahr. Im internationalen Vergleich liegt Deutschland (12,7 pmp) deutlich hinter den führenden Ländern wie Spanien (33,6 pmp), Österreich (25,9 pmp) und Belgien (25,2 pmp). Oft wird in diesem Zusammenhang die unterschiedliche rechtliche Grundlage in Deutschland (erweiterte Zustimmungslösung) und in Spanien, Belgien und Osterreich (Widerspruchslösung) herangezogen, wobei allerdings in Spanien in der Praxis ebenfalls nach der erweiterten Zustimmungslösung verfahren wird [2, 3].

Zusätzlich ist zu bemerken, dass ein bedeutender Teil der potenziellen Organspender (8–50%!) gar nicht entdeckt wird und somit schon vor der Abklärung medizinischer Kontraindikationen oder Ersuchen um Zustimmung der Angehörigen verloren geht [3].

Gegenwärtig werden jährlich etwa 800 LTx in der Bundesrepublik Deutschland in 24 Zentren durchgeführt, davon mehr als die Hälfte in den 4 Zentren Essen, Hannover, Berlin und Hamburg.

Weit über die Hälfte aller wartenden Patienten sind in diesen Zentren gemeldet. Sie alle sind abhängig von der Verfügbarkeit eines Spenderorgans, welches nach Richtlinien zur Organtransplantation gemäß §16 TPG zugeteilt werden, welche die Kriterien Blutgruppenkompatibilität, Dringlichkeitsstufen I–IV, Wartezeit, Konservierungszeit (kalte Ischämiezeit), Kinder und kombinierte Organtransplantation berücksichtigen.

Um den Pool der zur Verfügung stehenden Organe für die Patienten zu erhöhen und ihnen so rechtzeitig die Transplantation zu ermöglichen, wurden in den letzten Jahren verschiedene neue Techniken etabliert, wie z. B. die Teilleberspende- (Split-LTx) und die Lebendspender-LTx (living donor liver transplantation, LDLTx).

Seit 1989 hat sich die Split-LTx bei Kindern [4] und seit etwa 5 Jahren auch bei Erwachsenen schrittweise etabliert [5]. Kinder benötigen lediglich 25% des Lebervolumens eines Erwachsenen, manchmal sogar noch weniger. Hierzu wurde das Verfahren der Split-LTx entwickelt, wodurch die Transplantation von zwei Empfängern aus einer Leber möglich wurde [6]. Der Organmangel speziell für Kinder war anfänglich die Triebfeder, Eltern oder nahe Angehörige zur Spende eines relativ kleinen Teils der eigenen Leber zu bewegen. Die Entwicklung der Split-LTx hat dieses Vorgehen zum Teil relativiert, da nunmehr auch von Leichenorganen durch Entnahme des gleichen Lebersegments wie bei Lebendspendern – nämlich des linken lateralen Segments – eine Transplantation bei Kindern möglich wird.

Auf der technischen Basis der Split-LTx wurde anschließend die LDLTx für Kinder entwickelt [7]. Dieses Verfahren hat den entscheidenden Vorteil, die Wartezeit zu verkürzen, den Eingriff zu planen und über ein primär hervorragend funktionierendes Organ zu verfügen. Für diese Operation kommen aber nur Elternteilen in Frage, die einer gründlichen medizinischen und psychologischen Untersuchung für diesen Eingriff unterzogen wurden. Die Teilnahme der Eltern an dem Behandlungs- bzw. Heilungsprozess ihrer Kinder unter Inkaufnahme eines abschätzbaren Risikos steht heute weit mehr im Vordergrund als der früher existierende Organmangel. Mit den verfügbaren Methoden der Elterntransplantation oder der Leichenteil-LTx liegt die Mortalität von Kindern auf der Warteliste für LTx praktisch bei null [8].

Seit 5 Jahren wird als eine wesentliche Ergänzung zur Kinder-LDLTx die Erwachsenen-LDLTx durchgeführt, bei der ein kompletter Leberlappen, überwiegend der rechte (Segment 5–8), entnommen und präpariert werden muss [9]. Dieser Eingriff stellt für den erwachsenen Spender eine deutlich höhere Belastung dar als die Entfernung eines linken lateralen Segments für einen kindlichen Empfänger. Bei der Erwachsenen-LDLTx steht das Risiko des Eingriffs für den Spender im Vordergrund der Erwägungen und der Selektion. Auch unter den Erwachsenen sind der Wunsch und die Bereitwilligkeit zu einer Teilleberspende außerordentlich hoch, sodass Aufklärung und Untersuchung, ob der Spender für diesen Eingriff geeignet ist, besondere Bedeutung zukommen. Die Operation eines gesunden Individuums zum Zweck der Organspende ist für Nichtbeteiligte häufig nicht nachvollziehbar, wobei stets auf das wissentlich gefahrvolle Handeln seitens der Ärzte hingewiesen wird. Das Konzept des «primum nil nocere» (keinem Schaden zuzufügen) als ärztliche moralische Grundhaltung wird dabei kritisiert.

Im Kontext des Kranken und seines Umfelds stellt sich die Situation wesentlich anders dar, da die Möglichkeit der Lebensrettung eines nahe stehenden Menschen, d. h. der aktiv helfende Altruismus, möglich ist und konkret angestrebt werden sollte. Die Freiheit einer Entscheidung ist im Wesentlichen abhängig von Alternativmöglichkeiten, die von den behandelnden Ärzten ebenso angeboten werden müssen wie die Lebendspende selber.

Die Akzeptanz eines Risikos bei dieser Hilfsaktion ist unterschiedlich, sodass den behandelnden Ärzten an vorderster Stelle die Aufgabe einer Risikominimierung zukommt. Diese wird durch aufwändige Untersuchung und Beratungen erreicht, wobei etwa 80% aller potenziellen Spender für diesen Eingriff nicht geeignet sind. Allein deshalb wird die Häufigkeit der Leberlebendspende limitiert sein, wobei derzeit noch nicht zu sagen ist, welchen Stellenwert sie einnehmen wird.

Entscheidend für die Ergebnisse sind die Wahl des Operationszeitpunktes und die Indikationskriterien. Dabei sind 4 Indikationsgruppen zu unterscheiden:

1. Die elektive Indikation bei Patienten auf der normalen Warteliste, die eine Verkürzung der Wartezeit anstreben – möglicherweise sogar aus medizinischer Sicht warten könnten.
2. Patienten auf der Warteliste, deren Zustand sich von einer elektiven Indikation (Status 3, 2a) auf eine dringlichere Warteposition verschlechtert hat.
3. Patienten mit einer medizinisch-psychologisch begründeten Indikation, die aber aufgrund eines zu erwartenden eingeschränkten Überlebens des Organs (z. B. großes hepatozelluläres Karzinom in Leberzirrhose) keine Standardindikation darstellt.
4. Patienten aus dem Ausland, die von Allokativregeln ausgeschlossen sind und denen in ihrem Heimatland eine Nachsorge, aber keine Primärbehandlung zur Verfügung steht.

Die Komplikationen beim Spender stellen die wesentliche Kontraindikation zur breiten Anwendung der Leberlebendspende dar [10]. Die Komplikationen bei der linken lateralen LDLT sind deutlich gesunken und erlauben eine komplikationslose Operation bei 87% aller Eingriffe. Im Gegenteil dazu ist bei der rechtsseitigen Hemihepatektomie a priori mit einer hohen Morbidität zu rechnen, bedingt durch die technischen Anforderungen, die Dauer des chirurgischen Eingriffs und den Umfang des entnommenen Lebergewebes. Um eine vitale Bedrohung auszuschalten, bedarf es einer exakten Bestimmung der anatomischen Voraussetzungen und der Lebervolumina. Der Kompromiss darf nicht zu Lasten der Spender gehen, sodass sich häufig aufwändige Rekonstruktionen am Transplantat ergeben.

In Deutschland wurden im Jahr 2000 von den 780 LTx bereits 90 (11,5%) als LDLTx durchgeführt. Mehr als zwei Drittel davon fanden in den Zentren Essen, Hannover und Berlin statt.

Von April 1998 bis April 2002 wurden in der Klinik für Allgemein- und Transplantationschirurgie des Universitätsklinikums Essen insgesamt 373 Lebertransplantationen durchgeführt (Tab. 1, Abb. 2). Die derzeitigen Ergebnisse für das Patienten- und Transplantatüberleben nach LDLTx sind vergleichbar mit

Tab. 1. Anteil der verschiedenen LTx-Verfahren am Transplantationszentrum Essen zwischen April 1998 und April 2002

Verfahren	Anteil	
	n	%
Vollorgan-LTx	230	62
LDL-Tx	86	23
Split-LTx	52	14
Reduced-size-LTx	5	1
Gesamt	373	62

der konventionellen LTx und günstiger als bei der Split-LTx [5, 9].

Die LDLTx ermöglicht darüber hinaus, einem erweiterten Patientenkollektiv, d. h. Patienten, die aufgrund ihrer Grunderkrankung oder eines fortgeschrittenen Stadiums ihrer Erkrankung der konventionellen LTx nicht zuführbar sind, die potenziell kurative Therapie anbieten zu können. Hieraus resultiert zum einen, dass ein Patientengut mit einem erhöhten Risikoprofil operiert wird, zum anderen können durch die neuen Techniken aber auch bestimmte Patienten früher, d. h. in einem stabileren Stadium ihrer Erkrankung, operiert werden.

Die Definierung eindeutiger Selektionskriterien sowohl für den Spender als auch für den Empfänger werden weiter dazu beitragen, den Nutzen für den Spender zu maximieren und das Spenderrisiko zu reduzieren. Die Operation am lebenden Spender stellt einen erheblichen Eingriff dar, der tödliche Komplikationen in sich birgt, aber auch die Möglichkeit behandelbarer postoperativer Komplikationen zur Wiederherstellung der normalen Gesundheit. Neben der Erweiterung des Organpools hat diese Technik darüber hinaus den Vorteil einer höheren Qualität des zu transplantierenden Organs (im Vergleich zu den postmortal gespendeten Organen) und ermöglicht die LTx auch in Ländern, in denen aus religiösen Gründen keine postmortale Organspende stattfinden darf.

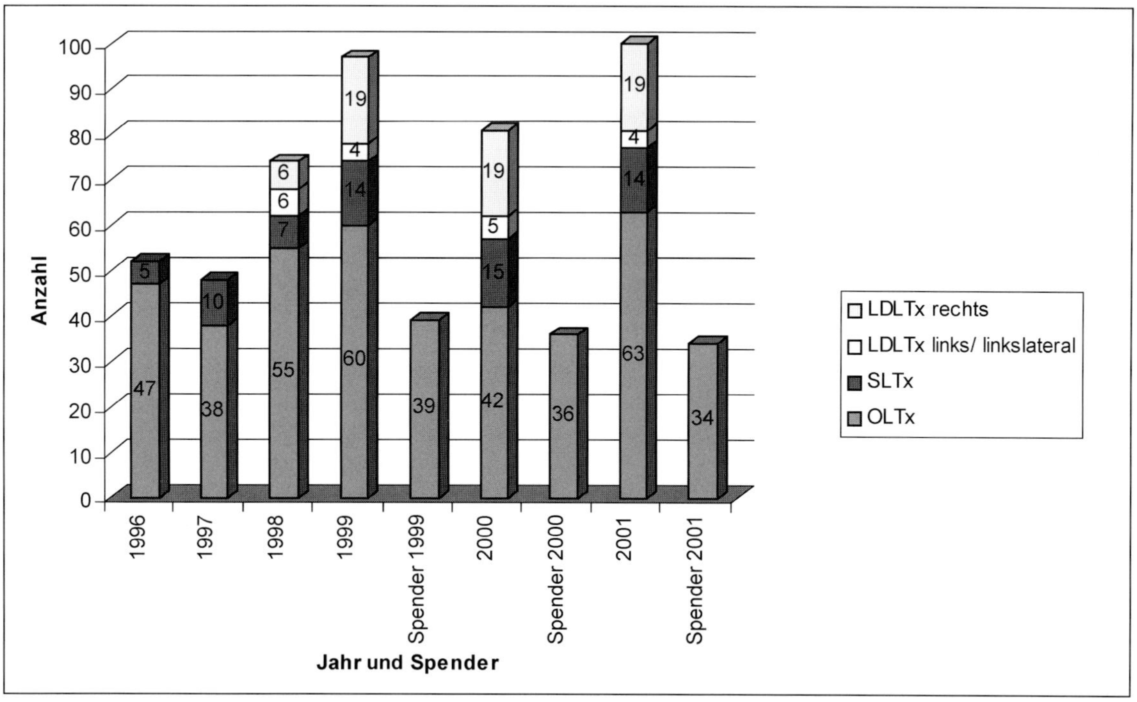

Abb. 2. Anzahl der LTx am Transplantationszentrum Essen.

Literatur

1 Deutsche Stiftung Organtransplantation (Hrsg): Organspende und Transplantation in Deutschland 1999. Neu-Isenburg, DSO, 2000.

2 Cohen B, Wight CA: European perspective on organ donation: Reaking down the barriers to organ donation. Transplantation 1999;68:985–990.

3 Gold SM, Schulz KH, Koch U: Der Organspendeprozess: Ursache des Organmangels und mögliche Lösungsansätze. Köln, Bundeszentrale für Gesundheitliche Aufklärung, Band 13, 2001.

4 Broelsch CE, Emond JC,Whitington PF, et al: Application of reduced-size liver transplants as split grafts, auxiliary orthotopic grafts, and living related segmental transplants. Ann Surg 1990;212:368–375.

5 Testa G, Malago M, Broelsch CE: Living-donor liver transplantation in adults. Langenbecks Arch Surg 1999;384:536–543.

6 Rogiers X, Malago M, Gawad K, et al: In situ splitting of cadaveric livers. The ultimate expansion of a limited donor pool. Ann Surg 1996;224:339–341.

7 Broelsch CE, Whitington PF, Emond JC, et al: Liver transplantation in children from living donors. Surgical techniques and results. Ann Surg 1991;214:428–437.

8 Broering DC, Mueller L, Ganschow R, Kim JS, Achilles EG, Schafer H, Gundlach M, Fischer L, Sterneck M, Hillert C, Helmke K, Izbicki JR, Burdelski M, Rogiers X: Is there still a need for living-related liver transplantation in children? Ann Surg 2001;234:713–722.

9 Broelsch CE, Malagó M, Testa T, Valentin-Gamazo C: Living donor liver transplantation in adults: Outcome in Europe. Liver Transplant 2000;6:S64–65.

10 Testa G, Malagó M, Nadalin S, Paul A, Frilling A, Broelsch CE: Complications and outcomes in adult living donor liver transplantation. Curr Opin Organ Transplant 2001;6:367–370.

Chirurgische Gastroenterologie Interdisziplinär

Chir Gastroenterol 2002;18(suppl 1):34–38

Nierenlebendspende

M. Zeier[a] M. Wiesel[b] J. Schweitzer-Rothers[c] M. Seidel-Wiesel[c] O. Hergesell[a] E. Ritz[a]

[a] Abteilung Innere Medizin I/ Sektion Nephrologie, Medizinische Universitätsklinik
[b] Sektion Nierentransplantation, Chirurgische Klinik, Abteilung Urologie
[c] Abteilung Medizinische Psychologie, Universität Heidelberg

Einleitung

Die Nierenlebendspende ist eine wichtige Maßnahme zur Erweiterung des Nierentransplantatangebots. Aktuelle Zahlen zeigen, dass trotz der gesetzlichen Regelung (Transplantationsgesetz) die Zahl der Organspender nicht zugenommen hat. Tabelle 1 vergleicht die Zahl der postmortalen Spendermeldungen und die tatsächlich realisierten Organentnahmen. Im Gegensatz dazu steigt die Zahl der Patienten auf der Warteliste für eine Nierentransplantation kontinuierlich an und liegt in der Bundesrepublik Deutschland aktuell bei 9490 (Eurotransplant 12 452) chronisch nierenkranker Patienten. Aufgrund des Spenderorganmangels hat die Nierenlebendspende in Deutschland zugenommen und liegt in vergleichbarer Höhe mit den durchschnittlichen Eurotransplant-Angaben (Tab. 2). Allerdings erreicht die Häufigkeit der Nierenlebendspende in Deutschland noch nicht diejenige in den Niederlanden oder Skandinavien.

Um bei einer geplanten Nierenlebendspende einen größtmöglichen Erfolg zu garantieren, muss sich sowohl der Nierenspender als auch der Empfänger in einem optimalen Zustand befinden. Auf die empfängerseitigen Untersuchungen kann hier nicht eingegangen werden. Zusammengefasst ist auf Risiken durch Gefäßerkrankungen, chronische bakterielle Entzündungen und chronische virale Infektionen, besonders die der Leber und bei Tumorerkrankungen, in der Vorgeschichte zu achten [1].

Tab. 1. Organspende in Deutschland 2000 (Quelle: Deutsche Stiftung Organtransplantation)

Spenderregion	Spendermeldungen	Realisierte Organspenden
Baden-Württemberg	290	121
Bayern	417	177
Mitteldeutschland	304	118
Norddeutschland	471	197
Nordostdeutschland	232	119
Nordrhein-Westfalen	425	159
Ostdeutschland	254	135
Deutschland gesamt	2410	1026*

* Rückgang um 1,25% im Vergleich zu 1999.

Tab. 2. Prozentualer Anteil der Nierenlebendspenden im Eurotransplant-Bereich. Vergleich 1990 und 1999

Länder	1990	1999
Belgien	3,5	5,4
Österreich	3,3	8,4
Deutschland	1,6	16,7
Niederlande	9,1	27,6
Eurotransplant gesamt	2,0	15,8

Die Voraussetzungen für die Nierenlebendspende sind vielschichtig und umfassen die medizinische Untersuchung, die psychologische Betreuung sowie soziale und juristische Aspekte.

Medizinische Grundlagen der Nierenlebendspende

Eine subtile Untersuchung des Nierenlebendspenders reduziert das Langzeitrisiko des Organspenders auf ein Minimum und garantiert gleichzeitig eine optimale Organqualität.

Lässt sich das Langzeitrisiko (Blutdruck, Nierenfunktion) eines Nierenlebendspenders eingrenzen?

Eine kürzlich vorgelegte Arbeit aus Stockholm [2] fand bei über 400 nachuntersuchten Nierenlebendspendern (durchschnittliches Alter zum Zeitpunkt der Nachuntersuchung 61 Jahre, Nachbeobachtungszeit 12 Jahre) keine Verschlechterung der Nierenfunktion, allerdings häufiger eine Hypertonie bei 30% der Spenderinnen und 50% der Spender (im Vergleich dazu Hypertoniehäufigkeit der entsprechenden Altergruppe von etwa 20%). Zusätzlich hatten 10% der Nierenlebendspender eine nachweisbare Proteinurie.

In einer früheren Untersuchung zeigte dieselbe Arbeitsgruppe, dass die Nierenlebendspende keinen Einfluss auf die Lebenserwartung des Nierenspenders hatte [3]. Eine weitere Studie dokumentierte eindrucksvoll, dass die große Mehrzahl der Nierenlebendspender die Organspende nicht bereuten [4]. Eine Untersuchung aus Minnesota an 57 Nierenlebendspendern, deren Uninephrektomie mehr als 20 Jahre zurücklag, ergab, dass die glomeruläre Funk-

KARGER

Fax +49 761 452 07 14
E-mail Information@Karger.de
www.karger.com

Accessible online at:
www.karger.com/journals/cga

Prof. Dr. Dr. h. c. mult. E. Ritz
Abteilung Innere Medizin I/Sektion Nephrologie
Universität Heidelberg
Bergheimer Straße 56 a
D-69115 Heidelberg (Deutschland)
Tel. +49 62 21-9 11 20, Fax -16 24 76

Tab. 3. Nierenfunktion und Blutdruck nach Nierenlebendspende an Hand des Heidelberger Spenderkollektivs (49 von 109 nachuntersuchten Spendern)

S-Kreatinin, mg/dl [1]	
Vor Spende	0,9 (0,7–1,3)
Klinikentlassung	1,2 (0,7–1,8)
Letzte Kontrolle	1,1 (0,9–1,7)
Blutdruck	
3 Spender > 140/90 mm Hg (bzw. Blutdruckmedikation) davon 1 Spender vor Nierenentnahme hypertensiv.	
Normale nächtliche Blutdruckabsenkung bei allen nachuntersuchten Spendern	

[1]Mediane Nachbeobachtungszeit 6 (1–13) Jahre.

tionsrate mit 82 ml/min zwar niedriger war als zum Zeitpunkt der Lebendspende (103 ml/min), im Vergleich zu gleichaltrigen Geschwistern (ohne Lebendspende, glomeruläre Filtrationsrate 89 ml/min) jedoch fast identische Werte hatte [5]. Die Ergebnisse unserer eigenen Nachuntersuchung an 109 Nierenlebendspendern sind in Tabelle 3 zusammengefasst.

Ältere Arbeiten weisen nach, dass der Verlust einer Niere auch langfristig kompensiert werden kann. In einer Untersuchung von Robitaille et al. [6] konnte nach Nephrektomie im Kindesalter nach einer Beobachtungszeit von 23 Jahren keine gehäufte Hypertonie oder Proteinurie bei normaler glomerulärer Filtrationsrate festgestellt werden. Selbst eine Zweidrittelresektion der Nieren (Tumor oder Tbc) ohne begleitende glomeruläre Erkrankung [7] führte zu keiner Progression der kompensierten Niereninsuffizienz.

Zusammenfassend ist daher das Risiko einer Nierenfunktionsverschlechterung minimal, wenngleich Blutdruck und Urinstatus sorgfältig überwacht werden sollten. Dies ist umso bedeutender, als das Transplantationsgesetz eine Nachsorge des Spenders zwingend vorschreibt und Lebendspenden nur dann zulässig sind, wenn die Spendernachsorge gewährleistet ist.

Auf welche medizinischen Risiken ist bei Nierenlebendspendern besonders zu achten?

Das Konzept der glomerulären Hypertonie spielt in der Spenderauswahl eine besondere Rolle. Glomeruläre Nierenerkrankungen wie Glomerulonephritis oder diabetische Nephropathie neigen nach einseitiger Nephrektomie besonders zu einer Progression der Niereninsuffizienz. Pathophysiologisch kommt es zu einer glomerulären Hypertonie. Der häufig erhöhte systemische Blutdruck wird durch ein infolge Uninephrektomie weitgestelltes Vas afferens in das erkrankte Glomerulum transmittiert und führt zu einem Glomerulosklerose mit Funktionsverlust. Hieraus ergibt sich, dass ein Diabetes mellitus definitiv ausgeschlossen sein muss. Ebenso darf keine diabetogene Stoffwechsellage (Abklärung durch oralen Glukosetoleranztest) vorliegen. Diabetogene Nierenschäden sind durch wiederholte Mikraltests, die ohne Befund sein müssen, und eine Glomerulonephritis durch Untersuchungen des Urinsediments (fehlende Hämaturie oder Proteinurie) auszuschließen. Im Zweifelsfall (z.B. wiederholt nachgewiesene mikroskopische Hämaturie) muss eine diagnostische Nierenbiopsie des Spenders gefordert werden. Im Rahmen unserer ambulanten Nierenlebendspenderuntersuchung konnten wir 2 Patienten mit dem Syndrom der dünnen Basalmembranen durch Biopsie identifizieren. Erwähnenswert ist der Befund, dass ein vierfach erhöhtes Risiko einer Nierenerkrankung beim verwandten Nierenlebendspender besteht [8]. In unserem Nierenlebendspenderprogramm ist 1 Fall von terminaler Niereninsuffizienz bekannt. Hier erfolgte die Nierenlebendspende bei manifestem Diabetes der Nierenspenderin.

Tab. 4. Checkliste für den potenziellen Nierenspender

Kriterium	Zu untersuchende Parameter
Nieren	S-Kreatinin, S-Harnstoff, Elektrolyte, Urinsediment, Mikroalbuminurie, Kreatinin-Clearance, 24-Stunden-Eiweißausscheidung, Nierensonographie
Blutdruck	24-Stunden-Blutdruckmessung falls Hypertoniker: Echokardiographie, Augenfundus, Intima/Mediadicke der A. carotis
Operative Planung	Angiographie, Magnetresonanzangiographie, Szintigraphie
Stoffwechsel	Blutzucker (nüchtern), HbA1c, Glukosebelastungstest
Blut	Serumchemie, Blutbild, Gerinnung
Immunologie	Blutgruppe, HLA-Typisierung, Crossmatch
Älterer Organspender	Tumorsuche

Besonderes zu beachten sind Familien mit hereditären Nierenerkrankungen (autosomal dominante polyzystische Nierendegeneration und Morbus Alport). Bezüglich der familiären Zystennieren gibt es heute klare sonographische Kriterien. Wenn nicht mehr als zwei Zysten je Niere im Alter von 30 Jahren sonographisch nachweisbar sind, ist der Nierenlebendspender mit hoher Wahrscheinlichkeit nicht Merkmalsträger [9]. Ein M. Alport des Nierenlebendspenders muss als wahrscheinlich gelten, wenn Hämaturie und/oder Proteinurie nachgewiesen wurden. Dieser Befund erfordert dann eine Nierenbiopsie (einschließlich Elektronenmikroskopie zur Feststellung der Basalmembrandicke) des Nierenlebendspenders.

Zusammenfassend muss eine bestehende Nierenerkrankung nach den heute anerkannten Methoden (Tab. 4) ausgeschlossen sein, um eine Nierelebendspende zu befürworten.

Wie ist im Falle einer essenziellen Hypertonie des potenziellen Nierenspenders zu verfahren?

Mit zunehmendem Alter ist auch eine Hypertonie des Nierenlebendspenders wahrscheinlicher [10]. Klinische und experimentelle Untersuchungen zeigen, dass die Veranlagung zum Bluthochdruck mit dem Nierentransplantat übertragen wird (Rettig, Curtis). Somit besteht nicht nur ein Risiko für den Spender, sondern auch für den Empfänger. Die Langzeitfunktion des Transplantats wird durch eine arterielle Hypertonie entscheidend beeinflusst [11]. Wir sind der Meinung, dass eine essentielle Hypertonie keine primäre Kontraindikation zur Nierenlebendspende darstellt. Allerdings muss durch eine 24-Stunden-Blutdruckmessung eine Normotonie mit nächtli-

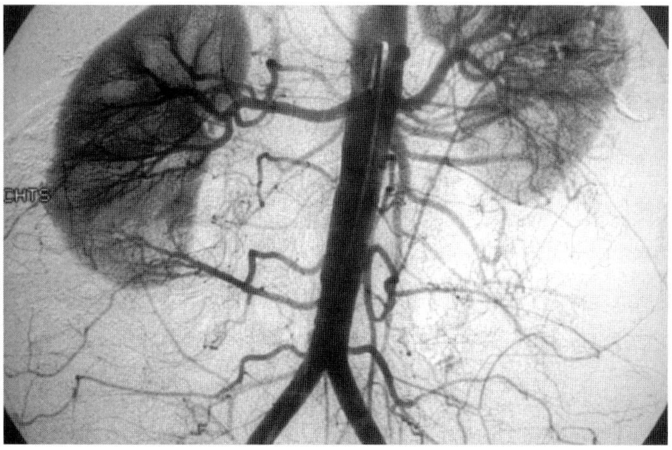

Abb. 1. Konventionelle Angiographie vor geplanter Nierenlebendspende.

cher Blutdruckabsenkung nachgewiesen sein [12]. Zusätzliche hypertoniebedingte Endorganschäden (Mikroalbuminurie, Intima/Mediadicke der Karotis, linksventrikuläre Hypertrophie) müssen ausgeschlossen werden. Der Spender ist zusätzlich über ein erhöhtes Risiko einer Verschlechterung der Hypertonie nach Uninephrektomie aufzuklären und entsprechend sorgsam zu überwachen.

Anatomische und funktionelle Gegebenheiten, die einen Einfluss auf die operative Strategie haben

Um das perioperative Risiko zu vermindern, sollten die Anzahl der Arterien und Venen bekannt sein. Hierzu kommt heute neben der konventionellen Angiographie die Magnetresonanzangiographie zunehmend zur Anwendung (Abb. 1, 2).

Die Szintigraphie mit seitengetrennter Clearance ist vor der Nephrektomie ebenfalls erforderlich, um Funktionsunterschiede beider Nieren zu erkennen. In jedem Fall muss die Niere mit dem höheren Funktionsanteil im Spender belassen werden. Falsche szintigraphische Ergebnisse sind bei einer Wanderniere (Absinken der Niere im Sitzen) oder bei doppelter Nierenanlage möglich und erfordern eine entsprechende Berücksichtigung.

Immunologische Voraussetzungen für eine Nierenlebendspende

Eine Voraussetzung für die Nierenlebendspende ist mit Ausnahme der Blutgruppe 0 die Blutgruppenkompatibilität. Eine Rhesusunverträglichkeit kann gelegentlich nach Transplantation zu einer leichten hämolytischen Anämie führen, hat jedoch nach unserer klinischen Erfahrung keine größere Relevanz. Auch bei der Lebendspende ist ein eindeutiger HLA-Effekt nachweisbar [13]. Neuere Untersuchungen zeigen jedoch, dass auch bei einer höheren Anzahl von HLA-Mismatches gute Langzeitergebnisse nach Nierenlebendspende zu erwarten sind [14]. Hier spielen sicher der Einfluss der kurzen Ischämiezeit und sehr wahrscheinlich auch eine ausgesuchte Spenderklientel (s. oben) eine wichtige Rolle. Ein negatives B- und T-Zell-Crossmatch vor einer geplanten Nierentransplantation sind ebenfalls erforderlich.

Gibt es den marginalen Nierenlebendspender?

Einzelne Arbeitsgruppen haben ein Lebendspendeprogramm von Organen der Großeltern auf ihre Enkel mit gutem Erfolg initiiert

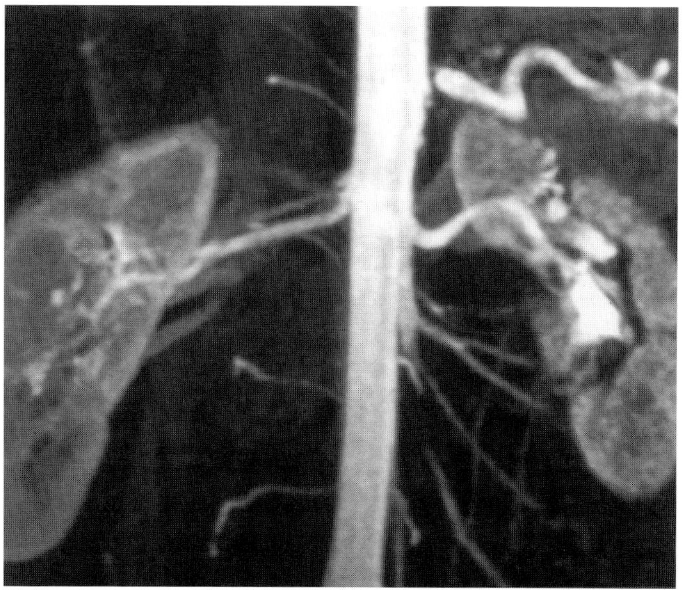

Abb. 2. MRT-Angiographie desselben Patienten vor Nierenlebendspende.

[15]. Tatsächlich verliert die Niere mit zunehmendem Alter nur wenig an glomerulärer Filtrationsrate [16] bei gleichzeitig erhaltener glomerulärer Reserve. Da die Niere des älteren Menschen eher ischämiesensibler ist, wirkt sich eine kurze kalte Ischämiezeit günstig auf die Funktionsrate nach Nierenlebendspende aus, wobei die kalte Ischämiezeit erwiesenermaßen eine wichtige Rolle für die Transplantatfunktion spielt [17]. Neben den üblichen Voruntersuchungen sollte jedoch die erhöhte Wahrscheinlichkeit eines unerkannten Malignoms und eines Diabetes mellitus im Alter bedacht werden. Deshalb muss die Abklärung eines Malignoms des Magen-Darm-Trakts, der Lunge oder der Prostata beim Mann bzw. des Uterus oder der Mammae bei der Frau vor einer Lebendspende erfolgen [18].

Chronische Viruserkrankungen und Nierenlebendspende

Der Zytomegalievirus(CMV)-Status des Nierenlebendspenders ist von größter Wichtigkeit. Da 60% der Organspender CMV-positiv sind, wird in vielen Fällen das Virus übertragen oder eine bereits bestehende Infektion reaktiviert. Besonders gefährdet ist der CMV-negative Empfänger einer CMV-positiven Niere. Durch entsprechende antivirale Prophylaxe können jedoch CMV-Virämie und -Erkrankung beim Empfänger reduziert werden [19]. Hepatitis-B- und -C-Virusträger und HIV-infizierte Patienten sind als Lebendspender ausgeschlossen.

Psychologische Aspekte einer Nierenlebendspende

Psychologische Aspekte einer Nierenlebendspende: das Heidelberger Beratungskonzept

Die Nierenlebendspende [20] scheint für Spender und Empfänger mehrheitlich einen positiven Einfluss auf die Lebensqualität zu haben. Untersuchungen berichten jedoch über 15–25% zum Teil er-

hebliche psychologische Probleme nach einer solchen Transplantation. Während die Beziehung Spender – Empfänger nach Transplantation meist noch besser und enger wird, gefährdet ein Transplantationsmisserfolg diese Beziehungsqualität: 4–10% der Spender bereuen ihren Schritt post hoc.
Bescheidene Erwartungen, insbesondere der Spender in Bezug auf den eigenen Lebensqualitätsgewinn, verbessern die Zufriedenheit nach Nierenlebendspende [21]. Postoperativ ist bei 15–20% der Empfänger mit meist depressiven Übergangskrisen zu rechnen.
Wir haben zur Prävention solcher kritischen Verläufe seit 1996 bei bislang 48 Spender-Empfänger-Paaren ein im Klinikalltag gut umsetzbares psychologisches Beratungskonzept entwickelt. Im ersten Schritt führen wir in der Abteilung für Medizinische Psychologie (ruhiges Sprechzimmer) zusammen mit den Transplantationsmedizinern (enge Kooperation zwischen Organmedizin und Psychologischer Medizin) gemeinsame Vorbereitungsgespräche für *alle* Spender- und Empfängerkandidaten (Ansatz der Systemischen Familienberatung) [22] *vor* der endgültigen Entscheidung durch. Thematisch nehmen die Vorbereitungsgespräche im Regelfall einen bestimmten Verlauf. Die Familiensituation wird an Hand des folgenden Genogramms ermittelt:

- Vorgeschichte des Umgangs mit der Krankheit
- Geschichte der Spendenidee, Bedenken und Zweifel
- Wünsche und Erwartungen
- Balance von Geben und Nehmen in der Beziehung
- realistisches Durchdenken von Komplikationen
- Geschichte und Stabilität der Beziehung
- offene medizinische Fragen
- Beratung kritischer Konfliktpunkte
- Angebot psychologischer Betreuung (auch nach der erfolgten Organspende bzw. Transplantation)

Die Gespräche sind ergebnisoffen. Im Zweifelsfall lehnen wir eine Transplantation nicht vollständig ab, sondern empfehlen «Nachdenkphasen» zur Klärung der deutlich gewordenen Konflikte.
Mit der postoperativen psychologischen Betreuung (oft 1–4 Gespräche) in Krisensituationen – häufig ausgelöst durch medizinische Komplikationen oder enttäuschte Erwartungen, symptomatisch meist als Angstzustände oder depressive Reaktionen – stehen wir bislang noch am Anfang.

Soziale und rechtliche Aspekte der Nierenlebendspende

Die sozialen Aspekte umfassen insbesondere die berufliche, wirtschaftliche und versicherungsrechtliche Sicherheit des Spenders. Da der Eingriff der Nierenlebendspende freiwillig ist, müssen diese Fragen mit den Krankenversicherungsträgern individuell besprochen werden. Der Nierenlebendspender ist ebenso darauf hinzuweisen, dass sich bei Lebensversicherungen die Versicherungsprämie möglicherweise erhöht bzw. bei Neuabschluss von Versicherungen hier Nachteile entstehen können. In jedem Fall ist es ratsam, die voraussichtliche Ausfallzeit dem Arbeitgeber mitzuteilen.
Die rechtlichen Aspekte der Nierenlebendspende sind im Transplantationsgesetz festgelegt und können hier im Detail nicht ausgeführt werden. Erwähnt werden soll die Vorstellung des Spenders vor einer Ethikkommission (ausführendes Organ: Bezirksärztekammern), um die Freiwilligkeit der Nierenlebendspende zu dokumentieren. Dies empfiehlt sich besonders im Fall von ausländischen Spender-Empfänger-Paaren (z. B. Sprachprobleme). Hier ist außerdem wichtig, dass der von der Ethikkommission bestellte Dolmetscher in keiner verwandtschaftlichen Verbindung zu dem Spender-Empfänger-Paar steht.
Eine Lebendspende kann aber nicht zuletzt nur dann erfolgen, wenn die Voraussetzungen für eine qualifizierte Nachsorge und die Bereitschaft für die Übernahme dieser Aufgabe gegeben sind.

Literatur

1 Zeier M, Ritz E: Preparation of the dialysis patient for transplantation. Nephrol Dial Transplant (in press).
2 Fehrman-Ekholm I, Duner F, Brink B, Tyden G, Elinder CG: No evidence of accelerated loss of kidney function in living kidney donors: results from a cross-sectional follow-up. Transplantation 2001;72:444–449.
3 Fehrman-Ekholm I, Elinder CG, Stenbeck M, Tyden G, Groth CG: Kidney donors live longer. Transplantation 1997;64:976–978.
4 Fehrman-Ekholm I, Brink B, Ericsson C, Elinder CG, Duner F, Lundgren G: Kidney donors don't regret. Transplantation 2000;69:2067–2071.
5 Najarian JS, Chavers BM, McHugh LE, Matas AJ: 20 years or more of follow-up of living kideny donors. Lancet 1992;340:807–810.
6 Robitaille P, Mongeau JG, Lortie L, Sinnassamy P: Long-term follow-up of patients who underwent unilateral nephrectomy in childhood. Lancet 1985;1:1297–1299.
7 Foster MH, Sant GR, Donohoe JF, Harrington JT: Prolonged survival with a remnant kidney. Am J Kidney Dis 1991;17:261–265.
8 Lei HH, Perneger TV, Klag MJ, Whelton PK, Coresh J: Familial aggregation of renal disease in a population-based case-control study. J Am Soc Nephrol 1998;9:1270–1276.
9 Papadopoulou D, Tsakiris D, Papadimitriou M: The use of ultrasonography and linkage studies for early diagnosis of autosomal dominant polycystic kidney disease (ADPKD). Ren Fail 1999;21:67–84.
10 Gasse C, Hense WH, Stieber J, Doring A, Liese AD, Keil U: Assessing hypertension management in the community: Trends of prevalence, detection, treatment, and control of hypertension in the MONICA Project. Augsburg, 1984–1995. J Hum Hypertens 2001;15:27–36.
11 Opelz G, Wujciak T, Ritz E: Association of chronic kidney graft failure with recipient blood pressure. Collaborative Transplant Study. Kidney Int 1998;53:217–222.
12 Ritz E, Schwenger V, Zeier M, Rychlik I: Ambulatory blood pressure monitoring: fance gadgetry or clinical useful exercise? Nephrol Dial Transplant 2001;16:1550–1554.
13 Hariharan S, Johnson CP, Bresnahan BA, Taranto SE, McIntosh MJ, Stablein D: Improved graft survival after renal transplantation in the United States, 1988 to 1996. N Engl J Med 2000;342:605–612.
14 Terasaki PI, Cecka JM, Gjertson DW, Takemoto S: High survival rates of kidney transplants from spousal and living unrelated donors. N Engl J Med 1995;333:333–336.
15 Nyberg SL, Manivel JC, Cook ME, Gillingham KJ, Matas AJ, Najarian JS: Grandparent donors in a living related renal transplant program. Clin Transplant 1997;11:349–353.
16 Fliser D, Zeier M, Nowack R, Ritz E: Renal functional reserve in healthy elderly subjects. J Am Soc Nephrol 1993;3:1371–1377.
17 Dragun D, Hoff U, Park JK, Qun Y, Schneider W, Luft FC, Haller H: Prolonged cold preservation augments vascular injury independent of re-

nal transplant immunogenicity and function. Kidney Int 2001;60:1173–1181.
18 Zeier M, Hartschuh W, Wiesel M, Lehnert T, Ritz E: Malignancy after renal transplantation. Am J Kidney Dis (in press).
19 Lowance D, Neumayer HH, Legendre CM, Squifflet JP, Kovarik J, Brennan PJ, Norman D, Mendez R, Keating MR, Coggon CL, Crisp A, Lee IC: Valacyclovir for the prevention of cytomegolovirus disease after renal transplantation. International Valacyclovir Prophylaxis Transplantation Study Group. N Engl J Med 1999;340:1462–1470.
20 Muthny FA, Koch U: Psychosoziale Aspekte der Nierentransplantation; in Koch U, Neuser J (eds): Transplantationsmedizin aus psychologischer Perspektive, Hogrefe, Goettingen, 1997, pp 61–81.
21 Schneewind KA, Ney B Hammerschmidt H, Oerter R, Pabst O, Schultz-Gambard E: Veränderungserwartungen und faktische Veränderungen der Lebensgestaltung bei Lebendnierentransplantation: Ein Vergleich zwischen verwandten und nicht verwandten Spender-Empfänger-Paaren. Transplantationsmedizin 2000;12;164–173.
22 v Schlippe A, Schweitzer J: Lehrbuch der systemischen Therapie und Beratung. Göttingen, Vandenhoeck und Ruprecht, 1996.

Chirurgische Gastroenterologie Interdisziplinär

Chir Gastroenterol 2002;18(suppl 1):39–41

Organ Donation after Cardiac Death

B. D. Shames A. M. D'Alessandro A. Krichevsky H. W. Sollinger

Department of Surgery, Division of Organ Transplantation, University of Wisconsin, Madison, WI

Introduction

There are currently over 79,000 patients on the waiting list for an organ transplant in the United States. However, UNOS reported that there were only 6,000 cadaveric organ donors last year in the United States and over 4,000 people died while on the transplant waiting list. This increasing disparity between potential recipients and donors has resulted in a renewed interest in retrieval of organs from non-heart-beating donors (NHBDs), now referred to as donation after cardiac death (DCD). DCD occurs when death is defined by the irreversible cessation of circulatory and respiratory functions. This is in contrast to standard heart-beating donors, in whom death is defined as irreversible cessation of all functions of the entire brain, including the brainstem. DCD can take place in a controlled or an uncontrolled setting. The controlled DCD is done through timing of withdrawal of life support and subsequent organ procurement. Uncontrolled DCD includes donors who have had a cardiopulmonary arrest shortly before arrival at the hospital and brain dead donors who suffer an unexpected cardiac arrest.

DCD is not a new concept; in fact, the first solid-organ transplants were from non-heart-beating donors [1]. In some countries where brain death is not accepted (Japan), DCD represents the only source of cadaveric donor organs. After the introduction of the Harvard Brain Death Criteria [2] the majority of transplant centers abandoned the use of DCD in favor of donation after neurological death (DND). Developments in organ procurement, organ preservation and immunosuppressive therapy have now allowed DCD to become a viable alternative to DND. However, the widespread reluctance to accept DCD as a source of organs is in part due to the warm ischemic insult sustained by the organs during procurement.

In 1997, the Institute of Medicine determined that the retrieval of organs from NHBDs was medically effective and ethically acceptable [3]. Further, in 1999 the Institute of Medicine recommended that all organ procurement organizations (OPOs) explore protocols for DCD. It is estimated that utilization of DCD could increase the number of organ donors by as much as 50% [4, 5]. At the University of Wisconsin, DCD has been utilized continuously since 1974. Initially only kidneys from these donors were used; however, since 1993 we expanded our program to include extrarenal organs from DCDs. This report summarizes our experience with DCD and reviews the current literature on this subject.

Organ Procurement and Preservation

We have previously published our technique of organ procurement in detail [6, 7]. Consent is obtained for organ donation as well as placement of femoral cannulas. The donor is brought to the operating room and the femoral artery and vein cannulas are placed using local anesthesia. The donor is then given 10,000–30,000 units of heparin and 10 mg of phentolamine to prevent thrombosis and vasospasm, respectively. A physician not associated with the transplant team, usually the patient's primary care physician, withdraws support. The actual organ procurement begins only after an additional 5 min elapsed after the declaration of death.

The procedure begins with the infusion of cold University of Wisconsin (UW) solution (Viaspan) into the femoral artery cannula while the femoral vein cannula is opened to gravity. A median sternotomy and midline abdominal incision are used and the intra-abdominal organs are removed en bloc [7]. On the back table, the portal vein, superior mesenteric vein, celiac artery, and renal arteries are flushed with additional UW solution and the organs are separated. This technique requires minimal in situ dissection, reduces operative time, and is compatible with the maximal utilization of all intra-abdominal organs [6].

From January 1993 to December 2001 we utilized a total of 73 controlled NHBDs. Of these 73 donors, 33 were kidney-only donors and 39 were considered for extrarenal donation. From the 39 multi-organ donors, 28 liver transplants and 25 simultaneous pancreas-kidney (SPK) transplants were performed. From 1 donor only the pancreas was procured [6, 8]. Tables 1 and 2 list the rationale for not transplanting livers or pancreases from NHBDs. Warm ischemic times ranged from 15 to 45 min [6]. Currently, our protocol is to retrieve extrarenal organs with up to 1 h of warm ischemia and to retrieve kidneys with warm ischemic times up to 2 h.

KARGER

Fax +49 761 452 07 14
E-mail Information@Karger.de
www.karger.com

Accessible online at:
www.karger.com/journals/cga

Hans W. Sollinger, MD
University of Wisconsin Hospital and Clinics, Department of Surgery
H5/701 Clinical Science Center, 600 Highland Avenue, Madison, WI 53792 (USA)
Tel. +1 608-262 8360, Fax -263 7652
E-mail hans@tx.surgery.wisc.edu

Table 1. Reasons for not transplanting livers from DCD

Reason	n
Severe steatosis	4
Centrilobular necrosis	1
Active hepatitis C	1
AB blood type with no recipient	1
Injured replaced right hepatic artery	1

Table 2. Reasons for not transplanting pancreases from DCD

Reason	n
Steatosis	4
Fibrosis	2
Diabetes	1
Pediatric	1
Nonretrieval	1

Table 3. Etiology of kidney loss after SPK

Etiology	n
Acute rejection	1
Chronic rejection	1
Death with functioning graft	1
Total	3

Table 4. Etiology of pancreas loss after SPK

Etiology	n
Late thrombosis	2
Acute rejection	1
Chronic rejection	1
Bleeding	1
Total	5

Kidney Transplantation from DCD

From 1974 to 1994, 897 renal transplants from NHBDs (554 pre-cyclosporine and 343 in the cyclosporine era) were performed at the University of Wisconsin [9]. Results from the cyclosporine era are reported here and compared with the 925 kidney transplants from heart-beating donors done in the same era. As expected, we have found that the initial function of kidneys retrieved from NHBDs is inferior to that of kidneys from heart-beating donors. Discharged creatinine was higher in the DCD group when compared with heart-beating donors (1.9 vs. 1.6 mg/dl, $p < 0.05$). Further, the incidence of acute tubular necrosis (ATN) and the need for dialysis was higher in the DCD group (19.5 vs. 12.1%, $p < 0.05$). However, long-term graft survival at 10 years was similar between DCDs and heart-beating donors (45.3 vs. 51.8%, p = not significant) [9].

An analysis of UNOS data compared early function and survival rates of 229 kidney grafts from NHBDs with those of 8,718 grafts from heart-beating donors [10]. The incidence of poor early function and need for dialysis in the 1st week after transplantation was higher in grafts from NHBDs compared with heart-beating donors (48 vs. 22%). Further, there was a higher incidence of primary nonfunction (PNF) in grafts from NHBDs (4 vs. 1%). Despite this poor early function, graft survival rates at 1 year were similar between the groups (83 vs. 86%) [10]. The 3% difference in graft survival occurred in the first 3 months after transplantation, and the authors suggest that this is related to ischemic damage of NHBD grafts [10]. The findings of poor early function and good long-term function of kidney allografts from NHBDs have been confirmed in multiple studies [4, 11–14]. Risk factors for poor early function and the need for dialysis appear to be inability to perfuse the organs prior to cardiac death, poorly perfused grafts, over 31 min of warm ischemic time, and more than 12 h of total ischemic time [15]. Further, donor age and the number of HLA-matched antigens had a minor influence on early graft function [15].

Pancreas Transplantation from DCD

Simultaneous pancreas kidney (SPK) transplantation has become the treatment of choice for patients with end-stage renal disease secondary to insulin-dependent diabetes mellitus [16]. We recently reported our experience with 18 initial SPK transplants from NHBDs [8] and have since done an additional 7 SPKs and 1 pancreas alone. Similar to the results with renal transplantation from NHBDs, the need for hemodialysis in the 1st week due to ATN was higher with SPKs from NHBDs than with SPKs from traditional heart-beating donors (22.2 vs. 4.1%, $p = 0.009$) [8]. No differences in pancreatic function were noted between NHBDs and heart-beating donors. All patients receiving SPKs from NHBDs became insulin-independent [8]. Despite a slightly higher incidence of rejection in the non-heart-beating group when compared to heart-beating donors, there was no difference in patient or allograft survival [8]. Causes of graft loss are shown in tables 3 and 4.

Our results as well as those from Japan [17] support the continued use of pancreas allografts from DCDs. Although the majority of experience has been with SPK transplantation, pancreas grafts from NHBDs could just as well be used for patients undergoing solitary pancreas transplantation [8]. Further, it is possible to isolate large numbers of islets from non-heart-beating donors, which can potentially be used as a source for islet cell transplantation [18].

Liver Transplantation from DCD

We recently reported our experience with liver transplantation from NHBDs [6]. This report included 19 liver transplants from NHBDs. We have performed 9 additional liver transplants from NHBDs since the publication of this manuscript. Patient survival in these 28 recipients is 68% (21/28) and graft survival 62% (21/33). Causes of graft loss are presented in table 5. No differences in hepatic artery, portal vein, or biliary complications have been noted when allografts from NHBDs were compared with standard heart-beating donors. However, the rate of PNF was higher in reci-

Table 5. Etiology of liver graft loss from DCD

Etiology	n
Death with a functioning graft	7
Primary nonfunction	2
Ischemic-type biliary stricture	2
Hepatic artery thrombosis	1
Sepsis	1
Total	13

pients of livers from NHBDs (10.5 vs. 1.3%, p = 0.04). The 2 cases of PNF occurred early in our experience with liver transplantation from NHBDs. Since that time we have instituted a protocol in which all recipients of NHBD livers receive intraoperative prostaglandin E, N-acetylcysteine, and vitamin E. Whether these agents have truly decreased our incidence of PNF is unclear; however, individually these antioxidants and membrane stabilizers are effective in preserving function [6].

Other centers have utilized livers from DCDs, although the overall experience is small and follow-up is short. The group from Albert Einstein Medical Center in Philadelphia recently reported their results with liver transplantation from NHBDs. They performed 8 liver transplants with grafts from NHBDs and have a 100% patient and graft survival at 18 ± 12 months of follow-up. Further, they had no poor graft function, PNF, arterial thrombosis or biliary complications [19]. The group from Pittsburgh reported on their experience with both controlled and uncontrolled DCD [20, 21]. Liver allografts from uncontrolled NHBDs had a 50% (3/6) incidence of poor function, while the 6 grafts from controlled NHBDs all had good initial function. The overall 2-year graft survival was 33%, and the 2-year patient survival was 58% [20, 21].

Conclusions

The overall results with organ transplantation from NHBDs have been successful. Despite a higher percentage of early graft dysfunction, the long-term function of kidney, pancreas, and liver allografts appears to be comparable to that of heart-beating donors. DCD should continue to be pursued as one way to help alleviate the current shortage of donor organs.

References

1 Starzl T, Marchioro TL, Brittain RS, Holmes JH, Wadell WR: Problems in renal homotransplantation. JAMA 1964;187:734–740.
2 A definition of irreversible coma: Report of the Ad Hoc Committee of the Harvard Medical School to examine the definition of brain death. JAMA 1968;205:337.
3 Institute of Medicine and National Academy of Sciences: Non-Heart-Beating Organ Transplantation: Medical and Ethical Issues in Procurement. Washington, D.C., National Academy Press, 1997.
4 Alvarez J, del Barrio R, Arias J, Vazquez S, Sanchez A, Iglesias J, Barra C, Ibarguren C: Non-heart-beating donors: Estimated actual potential. Transplant Proc 2001;33:1101–1103.
5 Kootrsa G: The asystolic, or non-heartbeating donor. Transplantation 1997;63:917–921.
6 D'Alessandro AM, Hoffmann RM, Knechtle SJ, Odorico JS, Becker YT, Musat A, Pirsch JD, Sollinger HW, Kalayoglu M: Liver transplantation from controlled non-heart-beating donors. Surgery 2000;128:579–588.
7 D'Alessandro AM, Hoffmann RM, Knechtle SJ, Eckhoff DE, Love RB, Kalayoglu M, Sollinger HW, Belzer FO: Successful extrarenal transplantation from non-heart-beating donors. Transplantation 1995;59:977–982.
8 D'Alessandro AM, Odorico JS, Knechtle SJ, Becker YT, Hoffmann RM, Kalayoglu M, Sollinger HW: Simultaneous pancreas-kidney (SPK) transplantation from controlled non-heart-beating donors (NHBDs). Cell Transplant 2000;9:889–893.
9 D'Alessandro AM, Hoffmann RM, Knechtle SJ, et al: Controlled non-heart-beating renal donation: A 21-year experience (Abstract). Am Soc Transplant Surgeons Annu Sci Meet, 1995.
10 Cho YW, Terasaki PI, Cecka M, Gjertson DW: Transplantation of kidneys from donors whose hearts have stopped beating. N Engl J Med 1998;338:221–225.
11 Nicholson ML: Renal transplantation from non-heart beating donors: Opportunities and challenges. Transplant Rev 2000;14:1–17.
12 Metcalfe MS, White SA, Saunders RN, Murphy GJ, Horsburgh T, Knight AJ, Nicholson ML: Long-term results of renal transplantation using organs from non-heart-beating donors. Transplant Proc 2001;33:826.
13 Hordijk W, Hoitsma AJ, van der Vliet JA, Hilbrands LB: Results of transplantation with kidneys from non-heart-beating donors. Transplant Proc 2001;33:1127–1128.
14 Metcalfe MS, Butterworth PC, White SA, Saunders RN, Murphy GJ, Taub N, Veitch PS, Nicholson ML: A case-control comparison of the results of renal transplantation from heart-beating and non-heart-beating donors. Transplantation 2001; 71:1556–1559.
15 Teraoka S, Nomoto K, Mito M, Yoshinaga K, Igata A, Sonoda T, Orita K, Fujimi S, Toma S: Multivariate analyses of factors contributing to early graft function in 759 kidney transplants from non-heart-beating donors. Transplant Proc 2001;33:1125–1126.
16 Sollinger HW, Odorico JS, Knechtle SJ, D'Alessandro AM, Kalayoglu M, Pirsch JD: Experience with 500 simultaneous pancreas-kidney transplants. Ann Surg 1998;228:284–296.
17 Tojimbara T, Teraoka S, Babazono T, Sato S, Nakamura M, Hoshino T, Nakagawa Y, Fujta S, Fuchinoue S, Nakajima I, Koike T, Abe M, Tomonaga O, Agishi T: Long-term outcome after combined pancreas and kidney transplantation from non-heart-beating donors. Transplant Proc 1998;30:3793–3794.
18 Clayton HA, Swift SM, Turner JM, James RF, Bell PR: Non-heart-beating organ donors: A potential source of islets for transplantation. Transplantation 2000;69:2094–2098.
19 Reich DJ, Munoz SJ, Rothstein KD, Nathan HM, Edwards JM, Hasz RD, Manzarbeitia CY: Controlled non-heart-beating donor liver transplantation. Transplantation 2000;70:1159–1166.
20 Casavilla A, Ramirez C, Shapiro R, Nghiem D, Miracle K, Bronsther C, Randhawa P, Broznick B, Fung JJ, Starzl T: Experience with liver and kidney allografts from non-heart-beating donors. Transplantation 1995;59:197–203.
21 Fung JJ: Use of non-heart-beating donors. Transplant Proc 2000;32:1510–1511.

Chirurgische Gastroenterologie Interdisziplinär

Chir Gastroenterol 2002;18(suppl 1):42–45

Kalte Ischämie und Konservierungsschaden: Was ist wirklich gesichert?

G. Otto

Transplantationschirurgie, Universitätsklinikum Mainz

Schlüsselwörter
Organkonservierung: kalte Ischämie, klinische Ergebnisse, Allokation

Zusammenfassung
Der Konservierungsschaden besitzt nach wie vor große klinische Bedeutung bei der Organtransplantation. Die kalte Ischämie ist einer der wesentlichen ätiologischen Faktoren. Nach jüngeren pathophysiologischen Vorstellungen ist eine Imbalance von Vasokonstriktion und Vasodilatation auslösender Faktor. Sie setzt eine Kaskade von Pathomechanismen in Gang. Die endotheliale Alteration als Ursache für die Mikrozirkulationsstörung lässt sich bereits bei der hypothermen Lagerung nachweisen. Eine verlängerte Dauer der kalten Ischämie führt zu einer Beeinträchtigung der Transplantatfunktion, die sich auch in geringeren Langzeitfunktionsraten niederschlägt. Trotz dieses Zusammenhangs kann eine patientenbezogene Allokation von Transplantaten nicht in Frage gestellt werden, da sie nur mit einer geringfügig längeren kalten Ischämiezeit verbunden ist.

Key Words
Organ preservation: cold ischemia, clinical results, allocation

Summary
Cold Ischemia and Preservation Damage: What is Really Reliable?
Preservation damage has been of great importance in clinical organ transplantation. Cold ischemia is one of the prinicipal pathomechanisms. Obviously, the imbalance between vasoconstriction and vasodilatation is the initiating mechanism which leads to a cascade of events. Morphological alterations can be observed as early as during hypothermic storage of the graft and are thought to be caused by the cold sensitivity of endothelial cells. Prolonged cold ischemia leads to graft dysfunction and in the long run to decreased graft survival. Nevertheless, the present patient-oriented organ allocation cannot be rejected for this reason since cold ischemia time is comparable to the time before implementation.

Primäre Nichtfunktion und Dysfunktion eines Transplantats sind noch immer wesentliche Komplikationen in der Transplantationschirurgie, obwohl eine unüberschaubare Zahl experimenteller und klinischer Untersuchungen sich des Problems angenommen hat. 6% aller Lebern und 6% aller Herzen werden wegen primärer Nichtfunktion retransplantiert, bei der Nierentransplantation sind es 2% [1]. Der Zustand des Organs vor der Entnahme, der Entnahmeprozess selbst, die Prozedur der Konservierung, die Art der Konservierungslösung, die Dauer der kalten Ischämie, die Rezirkulationsbedingungen und schließlich Faktoren beim Empfänger können Einfluss auf den Zustand des Transplantats nehmen.

Pathophysiologie des Reperfusionsschadens nach Ischämie

Es steht außer Zweifel, dass die Manifestation der Transplantatschädigung in erster Linie während der Reperfusion erfolgt. Die unmittelbar vorausgehende kalte Ischämie ist somit nur einer der ätiologischen Faktoren, die insgesamt zum Reperfusionsschaden führen, wenn auch zweifellos ein wichtiger. Seine Entstehung stellt sich nach der jüngeren Literatur wie folgt dar [2] (Abb. 1): Endotheliale Stickoxidsynthase und konstitutionelles Endothelin werden durch Schädigung, z. B. durch kalte Ischämie, aber auch unter warmer Ischämie, aus ihrem endothelialen Verbund freigesetzt und be-

KARGER
Fax +49 761 452 07 14
E-mail Information@Karger.de
www.karger.com

Accessible online at:
www.karger.com/journals/cga

Prof. Dr. G. Otto
Transplantationschirurgie
Universitätsklinikum Mainz
Langenbeckstraße 1, D-55101 Mainz (Deutschland)
Tel. +49 61 31 17-36 13, Fax -55 54
E-mail otto@transplantation.klinik.uni-mainz.de

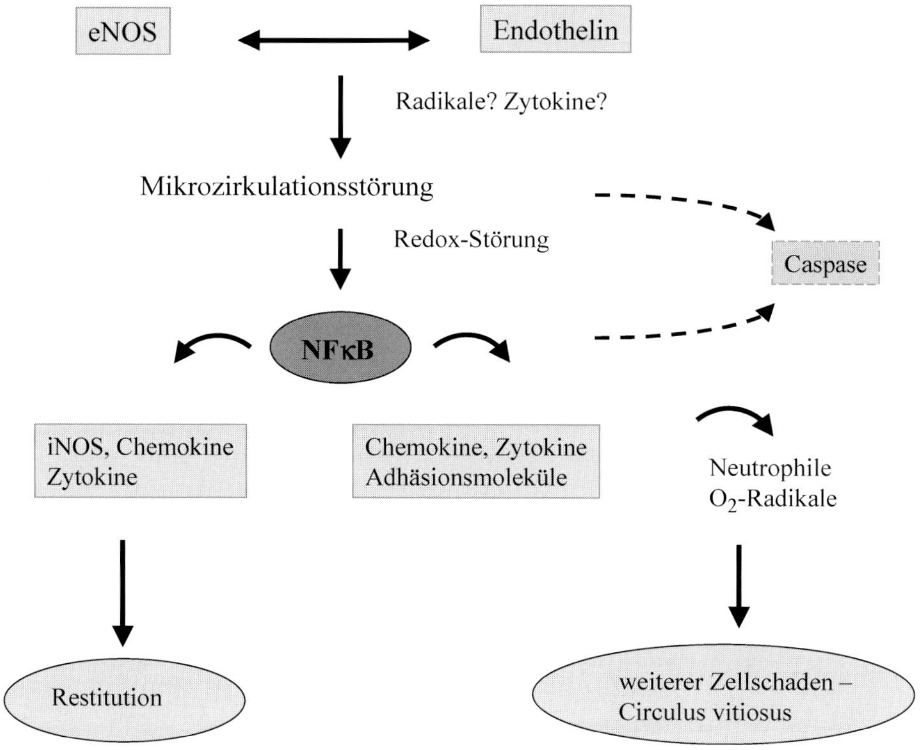

Abb. 1. Schematische Darstellung grundlegender pathophysiologischer Abläufe beim Zustandekommen des Ischämie-Reperfusionsschadens. eNOS = endotheliale Stickoxidsynthase; iNOS = induzierbare Stickoxidsynthase.

wirken eine Imbalance von Vasodilatation und -konstriktion, die zu Mikrozirkulationsstörung führt. Radikale spielen in dieser Phase der Schädigungskaskade möglicherweise noch keine Rolle. Die dadurch induzierte oder aggravierte Störung des Redox-Status des Gewebes bewirkt eine Aktivierung des NFκB, wodurch zahlreiche Mechanismen in Gang gesetzt werden. Wahrscheinlich erfolgt auch eine direkte Aktivierung von Adhäsionsmolekülen (ICAM, VCAM), wodurch weitere Mechanismen der Zelldestruktion, aber auch der Restitution, in Gang gesetzt werden (Radikale, Chemokine, Zytokine). Hierzu gehört ebenfalls die Apoptose.

Versuche, die Transplantatschädigung zu verringern, zielen meist auf Mechanismen ab, die Bestandteil dieser Kaskade sind. Die experimentellen Ansätze sind mannigfaltig. Modifikationen der Konservierungslösung und Änderungen des Perfusionsmodus (warme Flush-Perfusion, kontinuierliche Perfusion) lassen sich ebenfalls erst nach Rezirkulation beurteilen. Die Untersuchung biochemischer Parameter während der kalten Ischämie lässt kaum Rückschlüsse auf die Rezirkulationsphase zu. So wurden z. B. die Energiereserven der Zelle ausgiebig untersucht, wobei ihre Depletion nicht entscheidend für die spätere Organfunktion ist. Negative Einflüsse eines Konservierungsverfahrens lassen sich gut anhand der morphologischen Alterationen zeigen. Besonders deutlich sind sie während der Lagerungskonservierung der Schweineleber zu erkennen. Deren Sinusoide besitzen offenbar eine hohe Hypothermiesensibilität [3] (Abb. 2). Die Veränderungen sind hier so gravierend, dass bereits in dieser Phase der Konservierung eine Beeinträchtigung der Rezirkulation vorhersehbar ist. Es kommt zur fortschreitenden Destruktion bzw. Desquamation des Endothels, damit zu einer Denudierung des Dissé'schen Raums und zum Austritt von Hepatozytenbestandteilen (Blebs) [4, 5]. Die warme Rezirkulation bewirkt eine fulminante Progredienz dieser Schädigung. Ursächlich wird eine Kältesensibilität von Zytoplasmafortsätzen des Endothels angenommen, wodurch ein Detachment von darunter liegenden Hepatozyten zustande kommt.

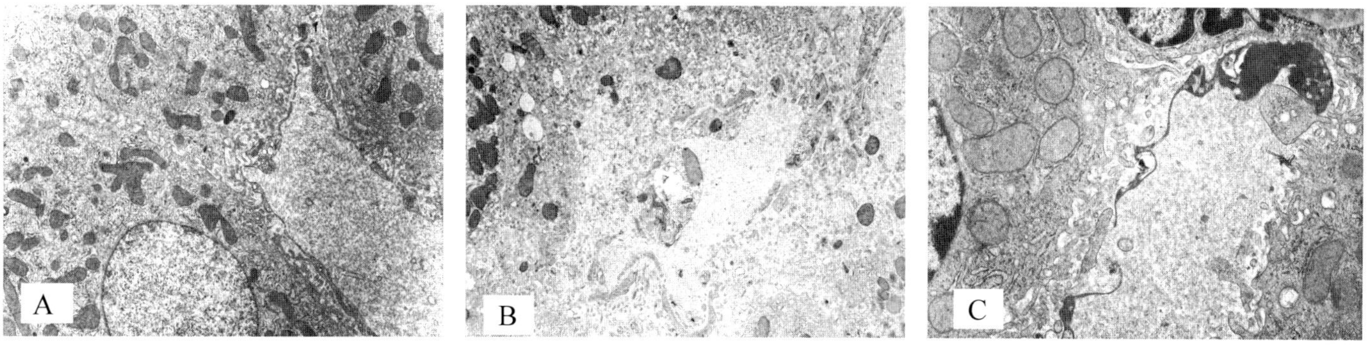

Abb. 2. Elektronenmikroskopie der sinusoidalen Schädigung bei hypothermer Lagerungskonservierung der Schweineleber mit Eurocollins. **A** Vor Lagerungsbeginn, **B** nach 6-stündiger Lagerung; klar erkennbare endotheliale Desquamation und Shedding von Zytoplasmabestandteilen, die (**C**) nach Reperfusion in ihrer Ausprägung zunehmen [3].

Kalte Ischämie und Transplantatfunktion

Die Folgen der Unterkühlung eines Organs wurden in jüngerer Zeit besonders eindrucksvoll in der Herzchirurgie gezeigt (Tab. 1). Die Endotheldicke nimmt unter Kardioplegie, besonders aber nach Rezirkulation, deutlich zu. Erst längere Zeit nach Rezirkulation normalisiert sich die Endotheldicke wieder. Die Einflüsse von Lagerungstemperatur und Zusammensetzung der Lösung sind offenbar äußerst komplex. Während unter normothermen Bedingungen die University-of-Wisconsin (UW)-Lösung als Konservierungslösung völlig versagt, ist sie bei langer hypothermer Lagerung anderen Lösungen überlegen (Tab. 2).

Tab. 1. Endotheldicke nach Ischämie-/Reperfusionsschaden im Verlauf der klinischen Herztransplantation [6]

Zeitpunkt	Endotheldicke, mm
Vor Kardioplegie	353 ± 21
Nach Kardioplegie	416 ± 71
30 min nach Transplantation	473 ± 45
1 Woche nach Transplantation	379 ± 39

Tab. 2. Herzkonservierung im Rezirkulationsmodell. Wiederaufnahme der Herzaktion (%) bei verschiedenen Konservierungszeiten und Temperaturen im Vergleich von St.-Thomas(ST)-, UW- und HTK-Lösung (n = 6/Gruppe) [7]

Lösung	Konservierungszeit, min/Temperatur, °C			
	35/37	120/20	300/4	450/1
ST	62,8	82,0	68,6	56,5
UW	–	46,8	66,2	70,6
HTK	–	41,4	47,2	43,0

Tab. 3. Ischämiezeit und Ergebnisse nach Lebertransplantation bei Konservierung mit UW-Lösung. Ergebnisse der Europäischen Multicenter-Studie

Transplantationen, n	315
Patienten, n	288
Primäre Dysfunktion, %	7,8
Primäre Nichtfunktion, %	7,4
Transplantatüberleben, %	
Nach 3 Monaten	
Sofortfunktion	91
Primäre Dysfunktion	58
Signifikanz	p < 0,001
Nach 6 Jahren	
Sofortfunktion	72
Primäre Dysfunktion	39
Signifikanz	p < 0,02
Kritische kalte Ischämiezeit, h	6

Der Einfluss der Dauer der kalten Ischämie auf die Integrität des Kapillarsystems konnte auch bei der klinischen Lebertransplantation gezeigt werden. Mittels Thermodiffusionsmessung ließ sich eine Korrelation von kalter Konservierungszeit und Abnahme der Mikrozirkulation nachweisen [8]. Eine kalte Ischämiezeit über 10 h führte bei 5 Patienten zur Retransplantation, während unter 10 h keine primäre Nichtfunktion auftrat. Der Unterschied war jedoch nicht signifikant. In der Europäischen UW-Multicenter-Studie mit 315 Lebertransplantationen bei 288 Patienten trat eine primäre Dysfunktion bei 7,8% und eine primäre Nichtfunktion bei 7,4% der Patienten auf. Die Dysfunktion war von hochsignifikantem Einfluss auf das Langzeitergebnis nach Lebertransplantation (Tab. 3). Aus der Studie ergab sich die Schlussfolgerung, dass eine kalte Ischämiezeit von 16 h eine kritische Grenze darstellt. In unserem eigenen Krankengut konnten wir keinen Einfluss der Konservierungszeit auf funktionelle Parameter oder das Transplantatüberleben nachweisen. Die Konservierungszeit lag jedoch durchweg unter 16 h. Die Korrelationskoeffizienten für die Maximalwerte innerhalb der ersten 10 Tage nach Transplantation betrugen für Bilirubin –0,57, GOT 0,03, GPT 0,1, gGT 0,04, alkalische Phosphatase –0,013 und Kreatinin 0,05.

Die Abhängigkeit der Langzeitergebnisse nach Organtransplantation ist auch in großen Sammelstatistiken für das Herz und die Leber nur marginal nachweisbar. Nach Nierentransplantation treten jedoch deutlichere Zusammenhänge zutage. In Abbildung 3 sind die 3-Jahres-Ergebnisse der Collaborative Transplant Study [10] für Herz-, Lungen-, Leber- und Nierentransplantation wiedergegeben. Die schlechteren Ergebnisse bei kurzen Konservierungszeiten (≤6 h) nach Nierentransplantation sind auf die bei dieser kurzen Konservierungszeit im Allgemeinen vernachlässigte HLA-Typisierung zurückzuführen. Konnte sie dennoch vorgenommen werden, so war sie auch in dieser Patientengruppe von großem Einfluss auf die Langzeitfunktion der Transplantate.

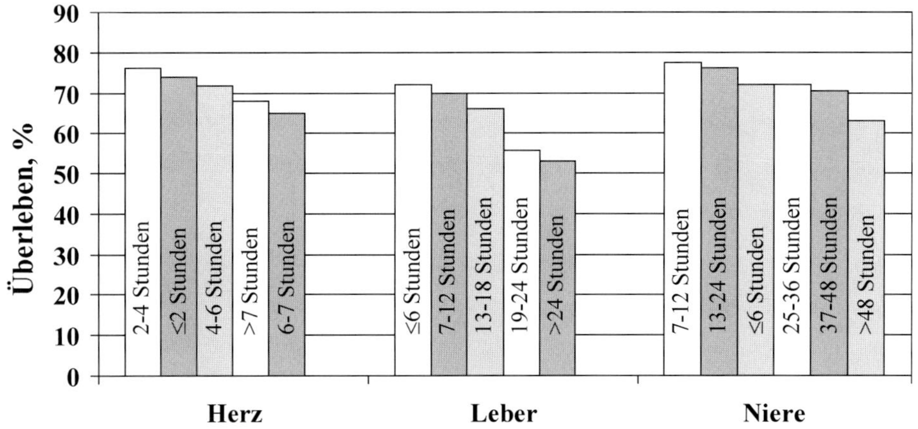

Abb. 3. 3-Jahres-Transplantatüberleben nach Herz-, Leber- und Nierentransplantation in Abhängigkeit von der kalten Ischämiezeit der Transplantate [10].

Kalte Ischämie und Organallokation

Bei der seit Juli 2000 in Deutschland und im Eurotransplant-Bereich gültigen Organallokation wird eine strenge, patientenbezogene Zuteilung der Organe vorgenommen. Dabei werden unter Umständen längere Transportwege des Organs notwendig, und es ist eine längere kalte Ischämiezeit zu erwarten. Tabelle 4 enthält die medianen kalten Ischämiezeiten für Leber, Herz und Niere vor und nach Einführung des neuen Allokationssystems [1]. Die Ischämiezeit hat bei Herz und Leber um 10%, dagegen bei der Niere nur minimal zugenommen. Mit Blick auf die Ergebnisse der Collaborative Transplant Study [10] liegen die Ischämiezeiten damit im gleichen Bereich wie vor Änderung der Allokation. Die gegenwärtige Allokation kann also nicht wegen einer inakzeptablen Zunahme der Ischämiezeiten in Frage gestellt werden.

Tab. 4. Kalte Ischämiezeit bei Herz-, Leber- und Nierentransplantation in Deutschland vor (2000) und nach (2001) Einführung der neuen Organallokation

Organ	Jahr	Transplantationen n	Analysierte Daten	Kalte Ischämiezeit (Median), h
Herz	2000	407	200	3,0
	2001	342	82	3,3
Leber	2000	691	442	8,2
	2001	572	324	9,0
Niere	2000	1871	1789	15,4
	2001	1689	1527	15,5

Schlussfolgerung

Die Dauer der kalten Ischämie besitzt fraglos eine Bedeutung für die Transplantatqualität. Eine Quantifizierung des Einflusses der kalten Ischämie und besonders die Wechselwirkung mit anderen Faktoren, die während dieser Periode bedeutsam sein könnten, gelingt bislang nicht. Auch der Einfluss anderer Faktoren, wie Fettleber, Spenderalter, Geschwindigkeit des Abkühlprozesses, Glykogengehalt der Leber, Osmolarität und Zusammensetzung der Konservierungslösung, ist somit nicht einschätzbar. Für jedes Organ wird eine zeitliche Limitierung der kalten Ischämie in der klinischen Praxis berücksichtigt. Diese Beschränkungen ergeben sich aus retrospektiven Daten, nicht jedoch aus fundiertem pathophysiologischem Wissen.

Literatur

1 Eurotransplant International Foundation. November 2001.
2 Inglott SF, Habib NA, Mathie RT: Hepatic ischemia-reperfusion injury. Am J Surg 2001;181:160–166.
3 Otto G, Wolff H, David H: Preservation damage in liver transplantation: Electron-microscopic findings. Transplant Proc 1984;16:1247–1248.
4 Caldwell-Kenkel JC, Currin RT, Tanaka Y, Thurman RG, Lemasters JJ: Reperfusion injury to endothelial cells following cold ischemic storage of rat livers. Hepatology 1989;10:292–299.
5 McKeown CMB, Edwards V, Phillips MJ, Harvey PRC, Petrunka CN, Strasberg SM: Sinusoidal lining cell damage: The critical injury in cold preservation of liver allografts in the rat. Transplantation 1988;46:178–191.
6 Koch A, Bingold TM, Oberlander J, Sack FU, Otto HF, Hagl S, Schnabel PA: Capillary endothelia and cardiomyocytes differ in vulnerability to ischemia/reperfusion during clinical heart transplantation. Eur J Cardiothorac Surg 2001; 20:996–1001.
7 Kumada Y, Yamamoto F, Ishikawa T, Kagisaki K, Shimada Y, Ohashi T, Ymamoto H, Hirose H: The temperature dependency of the protective properties of the St. Thomas' Hospital cardioplegic solution, the University of Wisconsin solution, and Bretschneider buffered solution. Nippon Kyobu Geka Gakkai Zasshi 1997;45:1954–1960.
8 Klar E, Angelescu M, Zapletal C, Kraus T, Bredt M, Herfarth C: Definition of maximum cold ischemia time without reduction of graft quality in clinical liver transplantation. Transplant Proc 1998;30:3683–3685.
9 Porte RJ, Ploeg RJ, Hansen B, van Bockel JH, Thorogood J, Persijn GG, Hermans J, Perpstra OT: Long-term graft survival after liver transplantation in the UW era: Late effects of cold ischemia and primary dysfunction. European Multicentre Study Group. Transpl Int 1998; 11:S164–S167.
10 Opelz G: Collaborative Transplant Study. Heidelberg, 2001.

Chirurgische Gastroenterologie Interdisziplinär

Chir Gastroenterol 2002;18(suppl 1):46–51

Bedeutung der Mikrozirkulationsstörung für die Manifestation des postischämischen Leberschadens

M. D. Menger B. Vollmar

Institut für Klinisch-Experimentelle Chirurgie, Universität des Saarlandes, Homburg/Saar

Schlüsselwörter

Ischämie · Reperfusion · Leber · Mikrozirkulation · Leukozyten-Endothelzell-Interaktion · Adhäsionsmoleküle · Apoptose

Zusammenfassung

Eine Vielzahl experimenteller Untersuchungen hat gezeigt, dass die Störung der nutritiven Mikrozirkulation von entscheidender Bedeutung für die Manifestation des postischämischen Reperfusionsschadens der Leber ist. Die Schädigung der Leber wird zum einen durch eine prolongierte Ischämie während der Reperfusion aufgrund des Ausfalls der sinusoidalen Perfusion (no-reflow), zum anderen durch eine ausgeprägte Entzündungsreaktion (reflow-paradox) mit Aktivierung von Thrombozyten, Granulozyten und Kupffer-Zellen verursacht. Der postischämischen sinusoidalen Perfusionsstörung liegen die Schwellung des Sinusoidendothels, die intravaskuläre Hämokonzentration sowie eine gestörte Balance zwischen den endogenen vasoaktiven Mediatoren Endothelin und Stickstoffmonoxid zugrunde. Die Antwort in Form einer Entzündung wird durch Freisetzung proinflammatorischer Mediatoren wie Tumornekrosefaktor-alpha, Interleukin-1 und Sauerstoffradikale, Hochregulation endothelialer und leukozytärer Adhäsionsmoleküle (Selektine, β-Integrine und ICAM-1) und Interaktion von Thrombozyten und Leukozyten mit dem mikrovaskulären Endothel vermittelt. Die daraus resultierende Parenchymschädigung beinhaltet – mit unterschiedlicher Ausprägung bei warmer und kalter Ischämie – sowohl den nekrotischen als auch den apoptotischen Zelltod, wobei die Bedeutung der Apoptose für die Gesamtschädigung der Leber noch nicht eindeutig geklärt ist. In klinischen Studien muss nun ermittelt werden, inwieweit neue Therapieansätze zur Protektion der postischämischen Mikrozirkulation die Ergebnisse nach großen leberchirurgischen Eingriffen mit vaskulärem Ausschluss bzw. nach Lebertransplantation verbessern können.

Key Words

Ischemia · Reperfusion · Liver · Microcirculation · Leukocytes – endothelial cell interaction · Adhesion molecules · Apoptosis

Summary

Impact of Microcirculatory Dysfunction on Manifestation of Postischemic Liver Injury

In hepatic ischemia-reperfusion, dysfunction of the microcirculation has to be considered as a primary step which triggers the final manifestation of tissue injury. Postischemic microcirculatory dysfunction includes the failure of sinusoidal perfusion, i. e., the no-reflow, which is caused by endothelial swelling, intravascular hemoconcentration, and a dysbalance between the vasoactive mediators endothelin and nitric oxide. Apart from perfusion failure, ischemia-reperfusion further promotes a microcirculation-associated inflammatory response (reflow-paradox), involving the release of aggressive mediators, such as oxygen radicals, tumor necrosis factor alpha and interleukin-1, the upregulation of leukocytic and endothelial adhesion molecules (selectins, beta-integrins, ICAM-1), and the interaction of platelets and leukocytes with the microvascular endothelium. Final parenchymal cell damage includes both necrotic and apoptotic cell death, which both may also represent a target for novel therapeutic strategies. Clinical studies have now to elucidate whether these strategies, which have been proven successful in the experiment, are capable of improving the final outcome of major liver surgery associated with ischemia-reperfusion, including liver transplantation.

KARGER

Fax +49 761 452 07 14
E-mail Information@Karger.de
www.karger.com

Accessible online at:
www.karger.com/journals/cga

Prof. Dr. M. D. Menger
Institut für Klinisch-Experimentelle Chirurgie
Universität des Saarlandes
D-66421 Homburg/Saar (Deutschland)
Tel. +49 6841 162 65-50, Fax -53
E-mail: exmdme@uniklinik-saarland.de

Einleitung

Bei einer Vielzahl chirurgischer Eingriffe an der Leber, wie die Versorgung nach Trauma [1, 2], die Resektion von Tumoren [3–5] und besonders die Transplantation [6, 7], ist der temporäre vaskuläre Ausschluss und damit die Induktion einer Ischämie unvermeidbar. Sowohl die Ischämie als auch die nachfolgende Reperfusion tragen zur Schädigung des Organs bei [8, 9]. Experimentelle Untersuchungen der letzten Jahre konnten zweifelsfrei nachweisen, dass die postischämische Beeinträchtigung der Mikrozirkulation einer Manifestation des parenchymatösen Gewebeschadens vorausgeht und gleichzeitig eine Determinante der reperfusionsassoziierten Leberdysfunktion darstellt [10, 11]. Die Beeinträchtigung der postischämischen Mikrozirkulation beinhaltet zum einen den Ausfall der nutritiven sinusoidalen Perfusion trotz globaler Reperfusion des Organs, zum anderen findet sich in Mikrogefäßen, welche nach Ischämie wiederperfundiert werden, eine Antwort in Form einer ausgeprägten Entzündung. Diese grundsätzlich unterschiedlichen Schädigungsmechanismen müssen sowohl bei der Analyse ihrer Pathophysiologie als auch bei der Entwicklung neuer Therapieansätze berücksichtigt werden.

Sinusoidales Perfusionsversagen

Mittels intravitaler Mikroskopie konnten verschiedenste experimentelle Untersuchungen nachweisen, dass prolongierte Ischämie zum Ausfall der Perfusion einzelner Sinusoide während der Reperfusion führen («no-reflow») [12, 13]. Auffälligerweise korreliert das Ausmaß der sinusoidalen Perfusionsstörung während der Reperfusion mit der Dauer der Ischämie [13] und beeinträchtigt entscheidend die Gewebeoxygenierung, die hepatozelluläre Integrität und die Parenchymfunktion [13–15]. Die kritische warme Ischämiezeit der Leber liegt bei 60 min und bewirkt einen Perfusionsausfall bei 15–30% der Sinusoide, wobei komplette azinäre Perfusionsausfälle nicht zu beobachten sind [13–15].
Im Gegensatz dazu zeigt eine 60 min dauernde warme Ischämie in Spendern mit nichtherzschlagenden Herzen (non-heart-beat doners, NHBD) bei Perfusion mit Konservierungslösung nicht nur massive sinusoidale Perfusionsausfälle von mehr als 50%, sondern auch ausgeprägte azinäre Durchblutungsdefizite [16]. Interessanterweise sind diese Defizite bei alleiniger aortaler Perfusion deutlich schwerwiegender als bei dualer, aortal- und portalvenöser Perfusion [16]. Des Weiteren ist das Defizit der azinären und sinusoidalen Perfusion in Lebern von NHBD bei Verwendung einer hochviskösen Konservierungslösung wie der University of Wisconsin(UW)-Lösung wesentlich stärker ausgeprägt als bei geringer viskösen Lösungen wie HTK [16, 17]. Die zusätzliche Verabreichung von Heparin und Phentolamin, nicht aber von Heparin allein, vermag diese ausgeprägten mikrovaskulären Perfusionsdefizite signifikant zu reduzieren [18]. Bei Verwendung der UW-Lösung zur Konservierung von NHBD-Lebern zeigt sich, dass eine Vorspülung mit Ringer-Laktat nicht ausreicht, um eine verbesserte mikrovaskuläre Äquilibrierung mit der Konservierungslösung zu erzielen, dass allerdings die zusätzliche Verabreichung von Streptokinase in der Lage ist, die mikrovaskuläre Perfusion mit Konservierungslösung entscheidend zu verbessern [17].
Nach Lebertransplantation, also nach kalter Ischämie und In-vivo-Reperfusion, lassen sich die kritischen Ischämiezeiten je nach verwendeter Konservierungslösung auf 8–24 h verlängern, die Charakteristika der Mikrozirkulationsstörung jedoch, d.h. azinäres und sinusoidales Perfusionsversagen, sind jenen nach warmer Ischämie vergleichbar [19, 20]. Eine zusätzliche warme Ischämie aufgrund intestinaler Kongestion in dem Fall, dass die Transplantation ohne portovenösen Shunt durchgeführt wird, verstärkt das Ausmaß der mikrovaskulären Perfusionsstörung nach Transplantation [21]. Das abrupte Aufwärmen des Transplantats bei In-vivo-Reperfusion mag ebenfalls zur Ausprägung der Mikrozirkulationsstörung beitragen. Aufgrund dessen kann das Vorspülen mit auf 37 °C angewärmter Ringer-Lösung oder Carolina rinse eine Protektion der Mikrozirkulation nach Transplantation bewirken [22, 23].
Der Pathomechanismus des postischämischen No-reflow beinhaltet die Schwellung sinusoidaler Endothelzellen und intravaskuläre Hämokonzentration [10, 11, 13]. Des weiteren können Leukozyten das sinusoidale Lumen okkludieren und damit die Perfusion blockieren. In der Tat zeigen die intravitalmikroskopischen Untersuchungen, dass nach Ischämie und Reperfusion die Anzahl der Leukozyten, die im sinusoidalen Lumen stagnieren, massiv ansteigt [24]. Die quantitative Auswertung dieser in Ruhe befindlichen Leukozyten zeigt jedoch , dass sie nur unwesentlich am postischämischen Perfusionsversagen der Sinusoide beteiligt sind, da die Mehrzahl der Sinusoide mit stagnierenden Leukozyten immer noch eine adäquate Perfusion aufweist [25].
Neuere Untersuchungen geben weiterhin den Hinweis, dass eine gestörte Balance der vasoaktiven Mediatoren Endothelin und Stickstoffmonoxid entscheidend zur postischämischen Mikrozirkulationsstörung der Leber beitragen [26]. Endothelin-1 scheint hierbei von besonderer Bedeutung zu sein, da die Verabreichung eines Endothelin-1-Antiserums die sinusoidale Konstriktion während postischämischer Reperfusion komplett verhindern und damit den Perfusionsausfall verringern kann [27]. Die Ergebnisse dieser ersten Untersuchungen von 1994 wurden in späteren Studien insoweit bestätigt, dass die Blockade von Endothelin signifikant die postischämische hepatische Mikrozirkulation durch Reduktion des sinusoidalen Perfusionsversagens verbessert [28–32], die Sauerstoffversorgung des Gewebes erhöht [29, 30] und die Leberschädigung, die Parenchymdysfunktion und die Mortalität vermindert [28, 29, 33]. Die Bedeutung des Gegengewichts von Stickstoffmonoxid in der Endothelin-Stickstoffmonoxid-Balance wurde dadurch nachgewiesen, dass die Blockade von endogen produziertem Stickstoffmonoxid während postischämischer Reperfusion den mikrovaskulären und hepatozellulären Schaden deutlich verstärkt [32, 34, 35]. Umgekehrt stellt die exogene Applikation des Stickstoffmonoxidspenders L-Arginin eine erfolgreiche therapeutische Option zur Verbesserung der Mikrozirkulation, der Gewebeoxygenierung und eine Verminderung der Funktionsbeeinträchtigung der Leber dar [36–38].

Mikrovaskuläre Leukozytenaktivierung

Obgleich die Wiederperfusion der Mikrogefäße nach einer länger andauernden Ischämie von vorrangigster Bedeutung für eine adäquate nutritive Versorgung des Gewebes ist, geht die Reperfusion dieser Gefäße paradoxerweise mit einer zusätzlichen Schädigung («reflow-paradox») einher. Die Aktivierung von Leukozyten (besonders neutrophile Granulozyten), ihre Adhärenz am mikrovaskulären Endothel sowie ihre transendotheliale Migration tragen in erheblichem Ausmaß zu dieser paradoxen Schädigung bei [39]. Dies wurde durch Experimente bestätigt, die aufzeigten, daß die Depletion der Leukozyten vor Ischämie erfolgreich den Reperfusionsschaden verhindern kann [40].

Intravitalmikroskopische Untersuchungen konnten weiter nachweisen, dass sowohl nach warmer [41] als auch nach kalter Ischämie [42, 43] Leukozyten in Sinusoiden, besonders aber in postsinusoidalen Venolen, mit dem mikrovaskulären Endothel interagieren. Die Tatsache, dass sich mit Hilfe eines monoklonalen Antikörpers gegenüber ICAM-1 (intercellular adhesion molecule-1) nicht nur die venuläre Leukozytenadhärenz signifikant reduzieren lässt, sondern auch die postischämische Leberfunktion und Parenchymintegrität verbessert werden können, belegt, dass die ICAM-1-mediierte Leukozytenadhärenz eine Determinante für den postischämischen Reperfusionsschaden darstellt [14]. Weitere Untersuchungen konnten bestätigen, dass auch Mac-1, der Ligand von ICAM-1 auf den neutrophilen Granulozyten, wesentlich für die Manifestation des leukozytenvermittelten Schadens benötigt wird [44, 45] und dass die Funktion von P- und L-Selektin, welche für den initialen Leukozyten-Endothel-Kontakt (Leukozyten-Rolling) erforderlich ist, ebenfalls zur Ausprägung der Gewebeschädigung beiträgt [46–49].

Mikrovaskuläre Plättchenaktivierung

Während der letzten beiden Jahre konnte mit Hilfe tierexperimenteller Studien gezeigt werden, dass auch die mikrovaskuläre Aktivierung von Blutplättchen an der Störung der Mikrozirkulation nach Ischämie und Reperfusion der Leber beteiligt ist [11, 50]. Die Plättchen adhärieren vornehmlich in den Sinusoiden, nicht aber in den postsinusoidalen Venolen [11]. Da die Plättchenadhärenz wahrscheinlich über P-Selektin vermittelt wird [50], sinusoidales Endothel jedoch P-Selektin nicht exprimiert [51], müssen die P-Selektinexpression und die Funktion der Blutplättchen selbst als die molekularen Mechanismen der postischämischen Plättchenadhärenz angesehen werden. Als Ligand auf dem sinusoidalen Endothel kämen dann Sialyl Lewis X und PSGL(P-selectin ligand)-1 in Frage; dies ist jedoch in weiteren Untersuchungen zu klären.

Die inflammatorische Antwort nach Ischämie der Leber beinhaltet also sowohl die Leukozyten- als auch die Plättchenaktivierung. Interessanterweise findet sich bei direkter Visualisierung dieser aktivierten Blutzellen in vivo eine auffällige Kolokalisation zellulärer Adhärenz in Sinusoiden [11]. Dies gibt Anhalt für einen gemeinsamen molekularen Signalweg in der Pathogenese der mikrovaskulären Adhärenz und lässt einen synergistischen Schädigungsmechanismus vermuten. In der Tat zeigen neueste Untersuchungen, dass Blutplättchen und Leukozyten synergistisch zum reperfusionsassoziierten Zelltod nach kalter Ischämie beitragen, und zusätzlich, dass Kupffer-Zellen in erheblichem Maße an der Vermittlung dieses Schadens beteiligt sind [52].

Kupffer-Zellaktivierung und proinflammatorische Mediatoren

Jaeschke et al. [53] konnten bereits 1991 zeigen, dass Kupffer-Zellen für die Induktion des oxidativen Stresses, für die Rekrutierung der Leukozyten und für das Priming der neutrophilen Granulozyten zur vermehrten Generierung von Sauerstoffradikalen über einen Complement-assoziierten Mechanismus verantwortlich sind. In der Tat zeigen intravitalmikroskopische Untersuchungen nach prolongierter kalter Ischämie, Transplantation und Reperfusion eine Aktivierung der Kupffer-Zellen mit massiver Steigerung ihrer Phagozytoseaktivität [54]. Entsprechend können durch Blockierung der Kupffer-Zellen, z.B. mit Gadoliniumchlorid, die CINC (cytokine-induced neutrophil chemoattractant) Freisetzung und damit die Leukozyteninfiltration reduziert [55, 56], die Mikrozirkulation verbessert [57] und schließlich die hepatozelluläre Schädigung vermindert werden [56]. Allerdings kann eine prolongierte Ischämiephase, insbesondere unter warmen Bedingungen, auch die Kupffer-Zellaktivität, wohl im Rahmen einer Immundepression, beeinträchtigen [58]. Unter diesen Bedingungen der Immuninkompetenz vermag dann die Restitution der Kupffer-Zellaktivierung über Immunstimulation die postischämische Leberschädigung und die damit zusammenhängende Letalität vermindern [59].

Das Reflow-Paradox und damit auch der postischämische Reperfusionsschaden müssen heute als Erkrankung in Form einer Entzündung angesehen werde. Die Stimulation von Kupffer-Zellen und Leukozyten bewirkt die Freisetzung einer Vielzahl von Entzündungsmediatoren einschließlich Sauerstoffradikalen und Zytokinen wie Tumornekrosefaktor-alpha und Interleukin-1 [10, 60]. Diese inflammatorischen Mediatoren aktivieren ihrerseits wieder endotheliale und leukozytäre Adhäsionsmoleküle, sodass ein Circulus vitiosus mit Aufrechterhaltung bzw. Verstärkung der Entzündung aufgebaut wird [61]. Die Bedeutung der proinflammatorischen Zytokine wird dadurch belegt, daß ihre Neutralisierung oder Blockierung die postischämische Leukozytenadhärenz und -infiltration sowie den Gewebeschaden effektiv reduziert [62, 63, 64–66]. Vergleichbar zeigt sich die Bedeutung der Sauerstoffradikale dadurch, dass nach Ischämie und Reperfusion 1. die Xanthinoxidaseaktivität und die radikalinduzierte intravaskuläre Hämolyse verstärkt sind [67], und 2. bei antioxidativer Behandlung mit Superoxiddismutase, Allopurinol oder N-Acetylcystein die Leukozytenadhärenz [67–69], der mikrovaskuläre endotheliale Schaden [70, 71] sowie die Leberfunktionsstörung vermindert sind [67–71]. Entsprechend konnte eine signifikante Protektion der Mikrozirkulation von Lebertransplantaten bei Verwendung von Konservierungs- und Ausspüllösungen mit antioxidativen Substanzen nachgewiesen werden [19, 22, 72, 73].

Apoptotischer Zelltod

Zweifelsfrei induzieren Ischämie und Reperfusion nekrotischen Zelltod. Jüngste Untersuchungen geben jedoch Hinweis darauf, dass der postischämische Reperfusionsschaden zu großen Teilen durch Apoptose sowohl von parenchymatösen als auch nichtparenchymatösen Zellen charakterisiert ist [74]. Während dies unter den Bedingungen von kalter und auch warmer Ischämie aufgezeigt wurde [74, 75], finden sich auch widersprüchliche Ergebnisse. Danach wird nach warmer Ischämie und Reperfusion der Leber dem apoptotischen Zelltod keine Bedeutung zugesprochen [76]. Eigene Untersuchungen mit einer neu etablierten In-vivo-Methode zur Detektion von apoptotischem Zelltod weisen nach warmer Ischämie und Reperfusion eine Rate von etwa 5–10% apopotischer Zellen auf, das größere Ausmaß an postischämischem Parenchymverlust wird jedoch durch Zellnekrose verursacht [77]. Bei kalter Ischämie und Reperfusion kann dem apoptotischen Zelltod eventuell größere Bedeutung zukommen [78].
Interessanterweise findet sich in In-vivo-Untersuchungen eine Kolokalisation von adhärenten Leukozyten, Blutplättchen und apoptotischen Zellen, welche eine kausale Bedeutung der Leukozyten- und Plättchenadhärenz für den apoptotischen Zelltod impliziert [11]. Erste Untersuchungen hierzu zeigen nun, dass in der Tat die P-Selektin vermittelte Blutplättchenadhärenz nicht unwesentlich zum postischämischen, reperfusionsassoziierten apoptotischen Zelltod nach kalter Ischämie beitragen [75].

Schlussfolgerungen

Der hepatische Ischämie/Reperfusionsschaden beinhaltet zwei pathophysiologische Entitäten, d. h. No-reflow und Reflow-paradox. Während das azinäre und sinusoidale No-reflow durch prolongierte Hypoxie die Gewebeschädigung verursacht, handelt es sich bei Reflow-paradox um eine Entzündung, welche über proinflammatorische Mediatoren, Aktivierung von Kupffer-Zellen und Rekrutierung von Leukozyten zur Beeinträchtigung der Leberfunktion beiträgt. Eine Vielzahl experimenteller Untersuchungen konnte in den letzten 5 Jahren neue Therapieansätze zur Verhinderung des Reperfusionsschadens erfolgreich etablieren. Diese Therapieansätze müssen nun in prospektiven klinischen Studien validiert werden.

Dank

Die Untersuchungen wurden durch die Deutsche Forschungsgemeinschaft (Me 900/1-2, Me 900/1-3 und Vo 450/7-1) gefördert. Frau Professor Brigitte Vollmar ist Heisenberg-Stipendiatin der Deutschen Forschungsgemeinschaft (Vo 450/6-1 und 6-2).

Literatur

1 Feliciano DV, Mattox KL, Jordan GL Jr, Burch JM, Bitondo CG, Cruse PA: Management of 1000 consecutive cases of hepatic trauma (1979–1984). Ann Surg 1986;204:438–445.
2 Pachter HL, Spencer FC, Hofstetter SR, Liang HG, Coppa GF: Significant trends in the treatment of hepatic trauma. Experience with 411 injuries. Ann Surg 1992;215:492–500.
3 Delva E, Camus Y, Nordlinger B, Hannoun L, Parc R, Deriaz H, Lienhart A, Huguet C: Vascular occlusions for liver resections. Operative management and tolerance to hepatic ischemia: 142 cases. Ann Surg 1989;209:211–218.
4 Huguet C, Addario-Chieco P, Gavelli A, Arrigo E, Harb J, Clement RR: Technique of hepatic vascular exclusion for extensive liver resection. Am J Surg 1992;163:602–605.
5 Vaillant JC, Balladur P, Nordlinger B, Karaitianos I, Hannoun L, Huguet C, Parc R: Repeat liver resection for recurrent colorectal metastases. Br J Surg 1993;80:340–344.
6 Ploeg RJ, D'Alessandro AM, Knechtle SJ, Stegall MD, Pirsch JD, Hoffmann RM, Sasaki T, Sollinger HW, Belzer FO, Kalayoglu M: Risk factors for primary dysfunction after liver transplantation – a multivariate analysis. Transplantation 1993;55:807–813.
7 Dousset B, Filipponi F, Soubrane O, Boillot O, Houssin D, Chapuis Y: Partial hepatic resection for ischemic graft damage after liver transplantation: a graft-saving option? Surgery 1994;115: 540–545.
8 Hasselgren PO: Prevention and treatment of ischemia of the liver. Surg Gynecol Obstet 1987; 164:187–196.
9 Huguet C, Gavelli A, Chieco PA, Bona S, Harb J, Joseph JM, Jobard J, Gramaglia M, Lasserre M: Liver ischemia for hepatic resection: where is the limit? Surgery 1992;111: 251–259.
10 Menger MD, Richter S, Yamauchi J, Vollmar B: Role of microcirculation in hepatic ischemia/reperfusion injury. Hepatogastroenterology 1999; 46:1452–1457.
11 Menger MD, Vollmar B: Role of microcirculation in transplantation. Microcirculation 2000;7:291–306.
12 Clemens MG, McDonagh PF, Chaudry IH, Baue AE: Hepatic microcirculatory failure after ischemia and reperfusion: improvement with ATP-$MgCl_2$ treatment. Am J Physiol 1985;248:H804–H811.
13 Vollmar B, Glasz J, Leiderer R, Post S, Menger MD: Hepatic microcirculatory perfusion failure is a determinant for liver dysfunction in warm ischemia-reperfusion. Am J Pathol 1994;145:1421–1431.
14 Vollmar B, Glasz J, Menger MD, Messmer K: Leukocytes contribute to hepatic ischemia/reperfusion injury via intercellular adhesion molecule-1-mediated venular adherence. Surgery 1995;117: 195–200.
15 Vollmar B, Glasz J, Post S, Menger MD: Role of microcirculatory derangements in manifestation of portal triad cross-clamping-induced hepatic reperfusion injury. J Surg Res 1996;60:49–54.
16 Richter S, Yamauchi J, Minor T, Vollmar B, Menger MD: Effect of warm ischemia time and organ perfusion technique on liver microvascular preservation in a non-heart-beating rat model. Transplantation 2000;69:20–24.
17 Yamauchi J, Richter S, Vollmar B, Menger MD, Minor T: Warm preflush with streptokinase improves microvascular procurement and tissue integrity in liver graft retrieval from non-heart-beating donors. Transplantation 2000;69:1780–1784.
18 Richter S, Yamauchi J, Minor T, Menger MD, Vollmar B: Heparin and phentolamine combined, rather than heparin alone, improves hepatic microvascular procurement in a non-heart-beating donor rat model. Transplant Int 2000; 13:225–229.
19 Marzi I, Walcher F, Menger M, Bühren V, Harbauer G, Trentz O: Microcirculatory disturbances and leucocyte adherence in transplanted livers after cold storage in Euro-Collins, UW and HTK solutions. Transplant Int 1991;4:45–50.
20 Post S, Menger MD, Rentsch M, Gonzalez AP, Herfarth C, Messmer K: The impact of arterialization on hepatic microcirculation and leukocyte accumulation after liver transplantation in the rat. Transplantation 1992;54:789–794.
21 Marzi I, Knee J, Menger MD, Harbauer G, Bühren V: Hepatic microcirculatory disturbances due to portal vein clamping in the orthotopic rat liver transplantation model. Transplantation 1991;52: 432–436.

22 Gonzalez A, Post S, Palma P, Rentsch M, Menger MD: Effects of warm Carolina rinse on microvascular reperfusion injury in rat liver transplantation. Transplant Int 1994;7:S155–S158.

23 Rentsch M, Post S, Palma P, Gonzalez AP, Menger MD, Messmer K: Intravital studies on beneficial effects of warm Ringer's lactate rinse in liver transplantation. Transpl Int 1996;9:461–467.

24 Vollmar B, Richter S, Menger MD: Liver ischemia/reperfusion induces an increase of microvascular leukocyte flux, but not heterogeneity of leukocyte trafficking. Liver 1997;17:93–98.

25 Vollmar B, Richter S, Menger MD: Leukocyte stasis in hepatic sinusoids. Am J Physiol 1996; 270:G798–G803.

26 Clemens MG, Bauer M, Pannen BH, Bauer I, Zhang JX: Remodeling of hepatic microvascular responsiveness after ischemia/reperfusion. Shock 1997;8:80–85.

27 Marzi I, Takei Y, Rücker M, Kawano S, Fusamoto H, Walcher F, Kamada T: Endothelin-1 is involved in hepatic sinusoidal vasoconstriction after ischemia and reperfusion. Transpl Int 1994; 7:S503–S506.

28 Dhar DK, Yamanoi A, Ohmori H, Nakashima Y, Yamamoto A, Osama NE, Kubota H, Kohno H, Nagasue N: Modulation of endothelin and nitric oxide: A rational approach to improve canine hepatic microcirculation. Hepatology 1998;28:782–788.

29 Mitsuoka H, Suzuki S, Sakaguchi T, Baba S, Miwa M, Konno H, Nakamura S: Contribution of endothelin-1 to microcirculatory impairment in total hepatic ischemia and reperfusion injury. Transplantation 1999;67:514–520.

30 Scommotau S, Uhlmann D, Löffler B-M, Breu V, Spiegel H-U: Involvement of endothelin/nitric oxide balance in hepatic ischemia/reperfusion injury. Langenbecks Arch Surg 1999;384:65–70.

31 Koeppel TA, Kraus T, Thies JC, Gebhard MM, Otto G, Post S: Effects of mixed ETA and ETB-receptor antagonist (Ro-47-0203) on hepatic microcirculation after warm ischemia. Dig Dis Sci 1997;42:1316–1321.

32 Pannen BH, Al-Adili F, Bauer M, Clemens MG, Geiger KK: Role of endothelins and nitric oxide in hepatic reperfusion injury in the rat. Hepatology 1998;27:755–764.

33 Urakami A, Todo S, Zhu Y, Zhang S, Jin MB, Ishizaki N, Shimamura T, Totsuka E, Subbotin V, Lee R, Starzl TE: Attenuation of ischemic liver injury by monoclonal anti-endothelin antibody, AwETN40. J Am Coll Surg 1997;185:358–364.

34 Wang Y, Mathews WR, Guido DM, Farhood A, Jaeschke H: Inhibition of nitric oxide synthesis aggravates reperfusion injury after hepatic ischemia and endotoxemia. Shock 1995;4:282–288.

35 Koeppel TA, Thies JC, Schemmer P, Trauner M, Gebhard MM, Otto G, Post S: Inhibition of nitric oxide synthesis in ischemia/reperfusion of the rat liver is followed by impairment of hepatic microvascular blood flow. J Hepatol 1997;27:163–169.

36 Jones SM, Thurman RG: L-arginine minimizes reperfusion injury in a low-flow, reflow model of liver perfusion. Hepatology 1996;24:163–168.

37 Shiraishi M, Hiroyasu S, Nagahama M, Miyaguni T, Higa T, Tomori H, Okuhama Y, Kusano T, Muto Y: Role of exogenous L-arginine in hepatic ischemia-reperfusion injury. J Surg Res 1997;69: 429–434.

38 Uhlmann D, Scommotau S, Witzigmann H, Spiegel HU: Exogenous L-arginine protects liver microcirculation from ischemia reperfusion injury. Eur Surg Res 1998;30:175–184.

39 Jaeschke H: Cellular adhesion molecules: regulation and functional significance in the pathogenesis of liver diseases. Am J Physiol 1997;273: G602–G611.

40 Jaeschke H, Farhood A, Smith CW: Neutrophils contribute to ischemia/reperfusion injury in rat liver in vivo. FASEB J 1990;4:3355–3359.

41 Vollmar B, Menger MD, Glasz J, Leiderer R, Messmer K: Impact of leukocyte-endothelial cell interaction in hepatic ischemia/reperfusion injury. Am J Physiol 1994;267:G786–G793.

42 Post S, Palma P, Gonzalez AP, Rentsch M, Menger MD: Timing of arterialization in liver transplantation. Ann Surg 1994;220:691–698.

43 Anthuber M, Farkas S, Rihl M, Menger MD, Schildberg FW, Jauch KW, Messmer K: Angiotensin-converting enzyme inhibition by enalapril: A novel approach to reduce ischemia/reperfusion damage after experimental liver transplantation. Hepatology 1997;25:648–651.

44 Jaeschke H, Farhood A, Bautista AP, Spolarics Z, Spitzer JJ, Smith CW: Functional inactivation of neutrophils with a Mac-1 (CD11b/CD18) monoclonal antibody protects against ischemia-reperfusion injury in rat liver. Hepatology 1993;17: 915–923.

45 Marubayashi S, Oshiro Y, Maeda T, Fukuma K, Okada K, Hinoi T, Ikeda M, Yamada K, Itoh H, Dohi K: Protective effect of monoclonal antibodies to adhesion molecules on rat liver ischemia-reperfusion injury. Surgery 1997;122:45–52.

46 Garcia-Criado FJ, Toledo-Pereyra LH, Lopez-Neblina F, Phillips ML, Paez-Rollys A, Misawa K: Role of P-selectin in total hepatic ischemia and reperfusion. J Am Coll Surg 1995;181:327–334.

47 Misawa K, Toledo-Pereyra LH, Phillips ML, Garcia-Cirado FJ, Lopez-Neblina F, Paez-Rollys A: Role of sialyl Lewis(x) in total hepatic ischemia and reperfusion. J Am Coll Surg 1996;182:251–256.

48 Palma-Vargas JM, Toledo-Pereyra L, Dean RE, Harkema JM, Dixon RA, Kogan TP: Small-molecule selectin inhibitor protects against liver inflammatory response after ischemia and reperfusion. J Am Coll Surg 1997;185:365–372.

49 Dulkanchainun TS, Goss JA, Imagawa DK, Shaw GD, Anselmo DM, Kaldas F, Wang T, Zhao D, Busuttil AA, Kato H, Murray NG, Kupiec-Weglinski JW, Busuttil RW: Reduction of hepatic ischemia/reperfusion injury by a soluble P-selectin glycoprotein ligand-1. Ann Surg 1998;227: 832–840.

50 Yadav SS, Howell DN, Steeber DA, Harland RC, Tedder TF, Clavien PA: P-Selectin mediates reperfusion injury through neutrophil and platelet sequestration in the warm ischemic mouse liver. Hepatology 1999;29:1494–1502.

51 Steinhoff G, Behrend M, Schrader B, Duijvestijn AM, Wonigeit K: Expression patterns of leukocyte adhesion ligand molecules on human liver endothelia. Lack of ELAM-1 and CD62 inducibility on sinusoidal endothelia and distinct distribution of VCAM-1, ICAM-1, ICAM-2, and LFA-3. Am J Pathol 1993;142:481–488.

52 Sindram D, Porte RJ, Hoffman MR, Bentley RC, Clavien PA: Synergism between platelets and leukocytes in inducing endothelial cell apoptosis in the cold ischemic rat liver: A Kupffer cell-mediated injury. FASEB J 2001;15:1230–1232.

53 Jaeschke H, Farhood A, Bautista AP, Spolarics Z, Spitzer JJ: Complement activates Kupffer cells and neutrophils during reperfusion after hepatic ischemia. Am J Physiol 1993;264:G801–G809.

54 Post S, Gonzalez AP, Palma P, Rentsch M, Stiehl A, Menger MD: Assessment of hepatic phagocytic activity by in vivo microscopy after liver transplantation in rat. Hepatology 1992;16: 803–809.

55 Hisama N, Yamaguchi Y, Ishiko T, Miyanari N, Ichiguchi O, Goto M, Mori K, Watanabe K, Kawamura K, Tsurufuji S, Ogawa M: Kupffer cell production of cytokine-induced neutrophil chemoattractant following ischemia/reperfusion injury in rats. Hepatology 1996;24:1193–1198.

56 Lentsch AB, Yoshidome H, Cheadle WG, Miller FN, Edwards MJ: Chemokine involvement in hepatic ischemia/reperfusion injury in mice: Roles for macrophage inflammatory protein-2 and Kupffer cells. Hepatology 1998;27:1172–1177.

57 Kukan M, Vajdova K, Horecky J, Nagyova A, Mehendale HM, Trnovec T: Effects of blockade of Kupffer cells by gadolinium chloride on hepatobiliary function in cold ischemia-reperfusion injury of rat liver. Hepatology 1997;26:1250–1257.

58 Vollmar B, Glasz J, Post S, Menger MD: Depressed phagocytic activity of Kupffer cells after warm ischemia-reperfusion of the liver. J Hepatol 1994;20:301–304.

59 Cursio R, Gugenheim J, Panaia-Ferrari P, Lasfar A, Tovey M, Chastanet S, Saint-Paul MC, Ferre C, Mouiel J: Improvement of normothermic rat liver ischemia/reperfusion by muramyl dipeptide. J Surg Res 1998;80:339–344.

60 Wanner G, Ertel W, Müller P, Höfer Y, Leiderer R, Menger MD, Messmer K: Liver ischemia and reperfusion induces systemic inflammatory response through Kupffer cell activation. Shock 1996;5:34–40.

61 Menger MD, Vollmar B, Glasz J, Post S, Messmer K: Microcirculatory manifestations of hepatic ischemia/reperfusion injury. Prog Appl Microcirc 1993;19:106–124.

62 Shibuya H, Ohkohchi N, Tsukamoto S, Satomi S: Tumor necrosis factor-induced, superoxide-mediated neutrophil accumulation in cold ischemic/reperfused rat liver. Hepatology 1997;26:113–120.

63 Shirasugi N, Wakabayashi G, Shimazu M, Oshima A, Shito M, Kawachi S, Karahashi T, Kumamoto Y, Yoshida M, Kitajima M: Up-regulation of oxygen-derived free radicals by interleukin-1 in hepatic ischemia/reperfusion injury. Transplantation 1997;64:1398–1403.

64 Colletti LM, Kunkel SL, Walz A, Burdick MD, Kunkel RG, Wilke CA, Strieter RM: The role of cytokine networks in the local liver injury following hepatic ischemia/reperfusion in the rat. Hepatology 1996;23:506–514.

65 Shito M, Wakabayashi G, Ueda M, Shimazu M, Shirasugi N, Endo M, Mukai M, Kitajima M: Interleukin 1 receptor blockade reduces tumor necrosis factor production, tissue injury, and mortality after hepatic ischemia-reperfusion in the rat. Transplantation 1997;63: 143–148.

66 Müller MJ, Vollmar B, Menger MD: Pentoxifylline reduces venular leukocyte adherence ('reflow-paradox') but not microvascular 'no-reflow' in hepatic ischemia/reperfusion. J Surg Res 1997;71:1–6.

67 Müller MJ, Vollmar B, Friedl HP, Menger MD: Xanthine oxidase and superoxide radicals in portal triad crossclamping-induced microvascular reperfusion injury of the liver. Free Radical Biol Med 1996;21:189–197.

68 Marzi I, Knee J, Bühren V, Menger M, Trentz O: Reduction by superoxide dismutase of leukocyte-endothelial adherence after liver transplantation. Surgery 1992;111:90–97.

69 Koeppel TA, Lehmann TG, Thies JC, Gehrcke R, Gebhard MM, Herfarth C, Otto G, Post S: Impact of N-acetylcysteine on the hepatic microcirculation after orthotopic liver transplantation. Transplantation 1996;61:1397–1402.
70 Nakano H, Nagasaki H, Barama A, Boudjema K, Jaeck D, Kumada K, Tatsuno M, Baek Y, Kitamura N, Suzuki T, Yamaguchi M: The effects of N-acetylcysteine and anti-intercellular adhesion molecule-1 monoclonal antibody against ischemia-reperfusion injury of the rat steatotic liver produced by a choline-methionine-deficient diet. Hepatology 1997;26:670–678.
71 Kondo S, Segawa T, Tanaka K, Izawa K, Hashida M, Kanematsu T: Mannosylated superoxide dismutase inhibits hepatic reperfusion injury in rats. J Surg Res 1996;60:36–40.
72 Post S, Rentsch M, Gonzalez AP, Palma P, Otto G, Menger MD: Effects of Carolina rinse and adenosine rinse on microvascular perfusion and intrahepatic leukocyte-endothelium interaction after liver transplantation in the rat. Transplantation 1993;55:972–977.
73 Post S, Palma P, Rentsch M, Gonzalez AP, Menger MD: Differential impact of Carolina rinse and University of Wisconsin solutions on microcirculation, leukocyte adhesion, Kupffer cell activity, and biliary excretion after liver transplantation. Hepatology 1993;18:1490–1497.
74 Kohli V, Selzner M, Madden JF, Bentley RC, Clavien PA: Endothelial cell and hepatocyte deaths occur by apoptosis after ischemia-reperfusion injury in the rat liver. Transplantation 1999;67: 1099–1105.
75 Sindram D, Porte RJ, Hoffman MR, Bentley RC, Clavien PA: Platelets induce sinusoidal endothelial cell apoptosis upon reperfusion of the cold ischemic rat liver. Gastroenterology 2000;118:183–191.
76 Gujral JS, Bucci TJ, Farhood A, Jaeschke H: Mechanism of cell death during warm hepatic ischemia-reperfusion in rats: apoptosis or necrosis? Hepatology 2001;33:397–405.
77 Schäfer T, Berrevoet F, Vollmar B, Scheuer C, Römer K, Menger MD: Reduction of apoptotic cell injury and inflammatory response after warm ischemia in rat liver by p53-inhibition with pifithrin-alpha (abstract). Eur Surg Res 2001;33:109.
78 Berrevoet F, Schäfer T, Vollmar B, Scheuer C, Römer K, Menger MD: p53-inhibition protects rat liver from cold preservation-induced apoptotic cell injury (abstract). Eur Surg Res 2001;33: 131.

Chirurgische Gastroenterologie Interdisziplinär

Chir Gastroenterol 2002;18(suppl 1):52–54

Spender-Empfänger-Konditionierung bei Organtransplantationen

A. L. Gerbes M. Bilzer

Medizinische Klinik II, Klinikum der Ludwig-Maximilians-Universität Großhadern, München

Konservierungsschäden tragen wesentlich zur primären Nichtfunktion bzw. Dysfunktion nach Lebertransplantation bei. Seit Etablierung der University-of-Wisconsin-Lösung haben sich keine neuen Verfahren zur Verhinderung des Konservierungsschadens in der Klinik durchsetzen können [1]. Verschiedene Substanzen sind in randomisierten klinischen Studien untersucht worden (Tab. 1).

Während die erste Studie zur Behandlung von Patienten nach Lebertransplantation für einen Zeitraum von bis zu 3 Wochen mit Prostagladin E1 eine Reduktion der Morbidität erbrachte [2], konnte dies in nachfolgenden Untersuchungen nicht bestätigt werden [3, 4]. Auch die Behandlung von Organspender bzw. -empfänger mit Prostaglandin I2 [5, 6], die Behandlung des Empfängers mit N-Acetylcystein [7–9] oder die Kombination von PGE1 und N-Acetylcystein [10] brachten keine eindeutig positiven Effekte. Diese Verfahren haben sich daher klinisch nicht durchgesetzt. Nachfolgend sollen drei Konzepte vorgestellt werden, mit denen am Klinikum der Ludwig-Maximilians-Universität in München versucht wird, klinisch umsetzbare neue Strategien zur Verhinderung des Konservierungsschadens zu etablieren. Diese basieren auf der Vorstellung einer Imbalance zwischen zytotoxischen Faktoren und endogenen Schutzmechanismen (Abb. 1). Die therapeutischen Ansätze zielen konsequenterweise auf eine Verminderung der zytotoxischen Faktoren bzw. eine Verstärkung endogener Schutzmechanismen.

Tab. 1. Randomisierte Studien zur Präkonditionierung bei der klinischen Lebertransplantation

Substanz	Studie	Vorteil
Prostaglandin E1	Henley et al., 1995 [2]	ja
	Klein et al., 1996 [3]	fraglich
	Neumann et al. 1998 [4]	nein
Prostaglandin I2	Klein et al., 1999 [5]	fraglich
	Neumann et al., 2000 [6]	nein
N-Acetylcystein	Bromley et al., 1995 [7]	nein
	Thies et al., 1998 [8]	fraglich
	Steib et al., 1998 [9]	nein
PGE1 und N-Acetylcystein	Bucuvales et al., 2001 [10]	nein

Erhöhung der extrazellulären antioxidativen Kapazität durch Glutathion

Aktivierte Kupffer-Zellen, die ortständigen Makrophagen der Leber, tragen insbesondere durch Freisetzung reaktiver Sauerstoffspezies wesentlich zum Reperfusionsschaden bei (Abb. 2). Maßnahmen zur Blockade von Kupffer-Zellen können daher tierexperimentell zur Reduktion des Reperfusionsschadens führen, erscheinen aber zum Einsatz in der Klinik wenig geeignet. Besondere Aufmerksamkeit unserer Bemühungen galt daher der Ent-

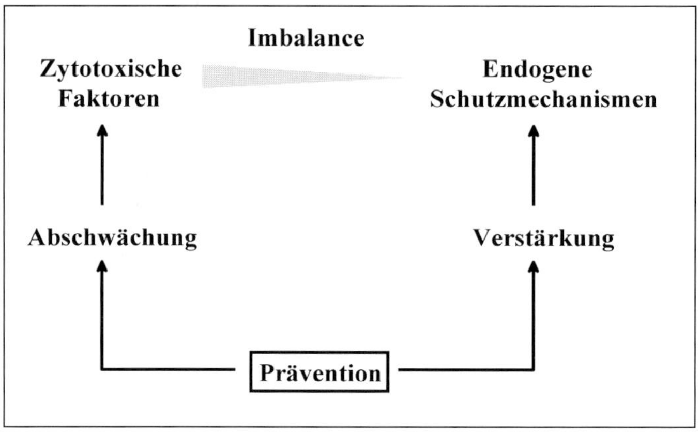

Abb. 1. Beeinflussung von Ischämie-Reperfusions-Schäden der Leber.

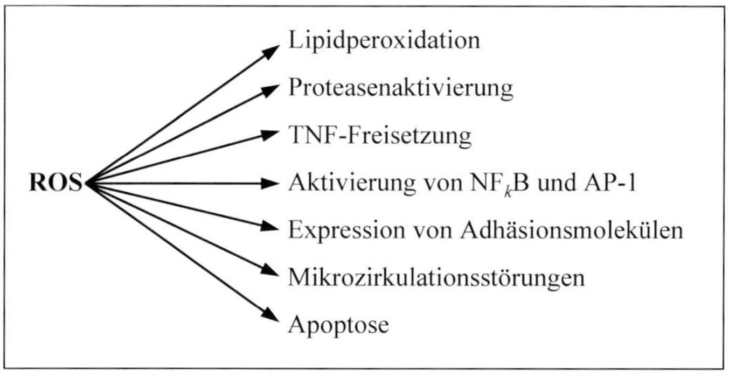

Abb. 2. Mechanismen der Zellschädigung durch reaktive Sauerstoffspezies (ROS) [modifiz. nach 1].

KARGER

Fax +49 761 452 07 14
E-mail Information@Karger.de
www.karger.com

Accessible online at:
www.karger.com/journals/cga

Prof. Dr. A. L. Gerbes
Medizinische Klinik II
Klinikum der Ludwig-Maximilians-Universität Großhadern
Marchioninistraße 15, D-81377 München (Deutschland)
Tel. +49 8 97 09 52-2 92, Fax -3 92

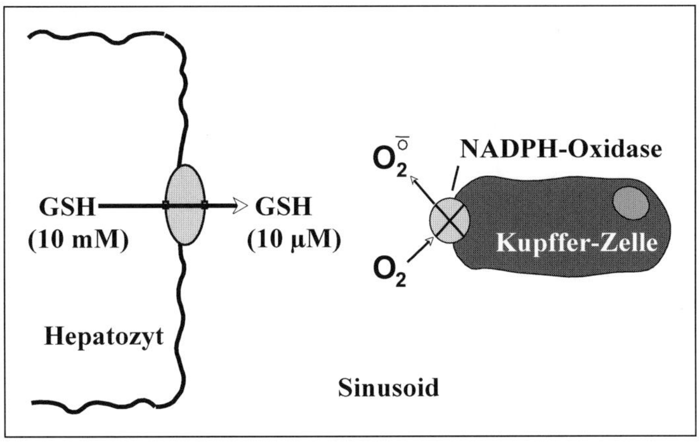

Abb. 3. Antioxidativer Schutz durch endogenes GSH [nach 1].

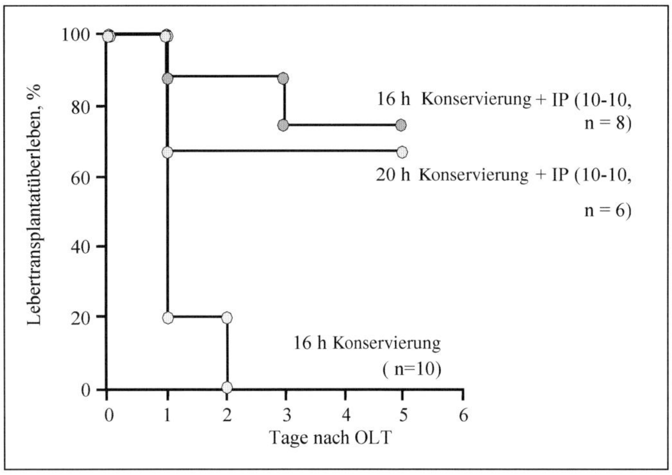

Abb. 4. Ischämische Präkonditionierung (IP) bei der Ratten-Lebertransplantation [nach 15]. OLT = orthotope Lebertransplantation.

wicklung protektiver Strategien, die vor den Folgen der Kupffer-Zellaktivierung schützen, ohne deren wichtige Abwehrfunktionen zu beeinträchtigen [11]. Von Hepatozyten freigesetztes Glutathion (GSH) kann dem oxidativen Stress der Kupffer-Zellen entgegenwirken [12], jedoch ist die extrazelluläre GSH-Konzentration im Sinusoidalraum im Vergleich zur intrazellulären sehr gering (Abb. 3).

Ausgehend von der Hypothese eines *extrazellulären Glutathionmangels* während der *Reperfusionsphase* untersuchten wir den Effekt einer Zufuhr millimolarer Glutathionkonzentrationen in der unmittelbaren Reperfusionsphase. Hierbei fanden wir eine deutliche Verringerung des hepatozellulären Schadens zusammen mit einer Verbesserung der Globalfunktion, gemessen am Gallefluss [13]. Dieser protektive Effekt ist auf eine Reduktion oxidativer Zellschäden durch aktivierte Kuffer-Zellen ohne Beeinflussung der Kupffer-Zellfunktion zurückzuführen [14].

Zusammen mit der guten Verträglichkeit von Glutathion beim Menschen und der guten Steuerbarkeit geben diese Befunde Anlass zur Durchführung einer prospektiven Untersuchung am Patienten.

Induktion endogener Schutzmechanismen

Ischämische Präkonditionierung

Ischämische Präkonditionierung wurde erstmals am Herzen als adaptive Antwort auf kurze Ischämieepisoden, die Zellschäden während einer nachfolgenden längeren Ischämie und Reperfusion vermindert, definiert. Experimentelle Untersuchungen hatten zeigen können, dass das Prinzip der ischämischen Präkonditionierung auch die Leber vor Reperfusionsschäden schützen kann. Bei der Rattenlebertransplantation konnte eine 10-minütige Ischämie, gefolgt von einer 10-minütigen Reperfusionsphase, den Konservierungsschaden nach 16- bzw. 20-stündiger kalter Lagerung erheblich reduzieren [15]. Während keines von 10 Tieren nach Transplantation einer über 16 h konservierten Leber mehr als 2 Tage überlebte, war dies bei 8 von 10 Tieren nach ischämischer Präkonditionierung der Fall (Abb. 4).

Interessanterweise schützt die ischämische Präkonditionierung auch gegen oxidativen Stress durch direkte Zufuhr von Wasserstoffperoxid, ohne andererseits die Produktion reaktiver Sauerstoffspezies durch Kupffer-Zellen zu beeinträchtigen [16]. Die protektiven Effekte der ischämischen Präkonditionierung werden auf Adenosinrezeptor vermittelte Stimulation der Stickstoffmonoxidbildung zurückgeführt. Letztere führt über Aktivierung der löslichen Guanylatcyclase zur Bildung des Second-messengers cyclisches Guanosinmonophosphat (cGMP). Dies legte die Suche nach einer gezielten pharmakologischen Stimulation der cGMP-Bildung nahe.

Hormonelle Präkonditionierung mit atrialem natriuretischem Peptid

Atriales natriuretisches Peptid (ANP) wird physiologischerweise von Myozyten des Herzvorhofs gebildet. Durch Stimulation der partikulären Guanylatcyclase führt es zur Erhöhung des intrazellulären cGMP-Gehalts. In der Tat schützte eine 20-minütige präischämische Gabe von 200 nM ANP die Leber vor Reperfusionsschäden nach warmer wie kalter Ischämie. Ähnliche Effekte konnten durch Gabe des Second-messengers 8-Br-cGMP erzielt werden, ein Hinweis auf die Rezeptor vermittelte Wirkung von ANP [17]. Hierdurch kommt es zur pharmakologischen Aktivierung von Hitzeschockproteinen [18].

In weiteren Untersuchungen konnten wir zeigen, dass ANP vor der oxidativen Schädigung durch aktivierte Kupffer-Zellen schützt [19]. Hierfür ist nicht eine Beeinflussung der Radikalproduktion durch Kupffer-Zellen verantwortlich, sondern eine zelluläre Resistenz gegenüber reaktiven Sauerstoffspezies (Abb. 5).

Ähnlich wie bei der ischämischen Präkonditionierung handelt es sich wiederum um die Induktion endogener Schutzmechanismen. Bei der hormonellen und ischämischen Präkonditionierung ergeben sich also Parallelen hinsichtlich der durch cGMP vermittelten Resistenz gegenüber reaktiven Sauerstoffspezies (Abb. 6).

Die Charakterisierung der durch cGMP induzierten endogenen Schutzmechanismen ist Ziel weiterer Untersuchungen.

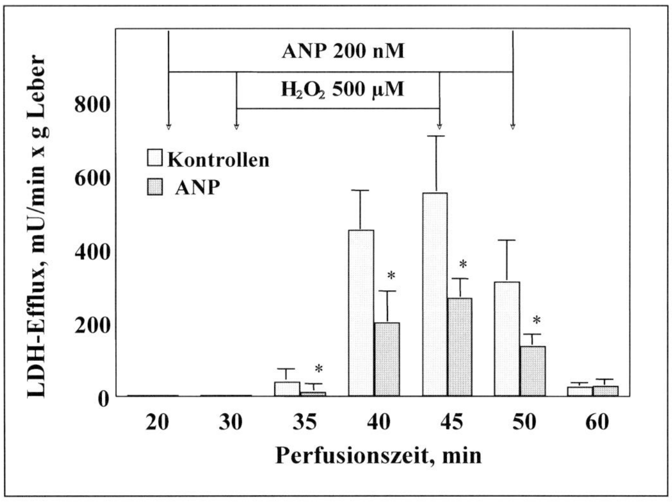

Abb. 5. Prävention oxidativer Zellschäden durch ANP [nach 19]. * p = 0,05 Versuskontrollen.

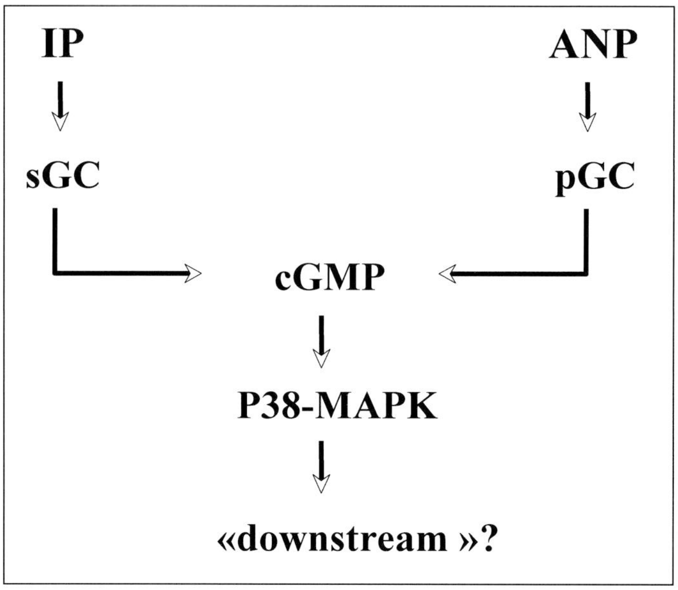

Abb. 6. Mechanismen der ischämischen und hormonellen Präkonditionierung.

Literatur

1 Bilzer M, Gerbes AL: Preservation injury of the liver: Mechanisms and novel therapeutic strategies. J Hepatol 2000:32:580–515.

2 Henley KS, Lucey MR, Normolle DP, Merion RM, McLaren ID, Crider BA, Mackie DS, Shieck VL, Nostrant TT, Brown KA et al: A double-blind, randomized, placebo-controlled trial of prostaglandin E1 in liver transplantation. Hepatology 1995;21:366–372.

3 Klein AS, Cofer JB, Pruett TL, Thuluvath PJ, McGory R, Uber L, Stevenson WC, Baliga P, Burdick JF: Prostaglandin E1 administration following orthotopic liver transplantation: A randomized prospective multicenter trial. Gastroenterology 1996;111:710–715.

4 Neumann UP, Kaisers U, Langrehr JM, Lang M, Glanemann M, Raakow R, Steinmuller T, Settmacher U, Muller AR, Bechstein WO, Neuhaus P: Treatment with PGE1 in patients after liver transplantation. Transplant Proc 1998;30: 1869–1870.

5 Klein M, Geoghegan J, Wangemann R, Bockler D, Schmidt K, Scheele J: Preconditioning of donor livers with prostaglandin I2 before retrieval decreases hepatocellular ischemia-reperfusion injury. Transplantation 1999;67:1128–1132.

6 Neumann UP, Kaisers U, Langrehr JM, Glanemann M, Muller AR, Lang M, Jorres A, Settmacher U, Bechstein WO, Neuhaus P: Administration of prostacyclin after liver transplantation: A placebo controlled randomized trial. Clin Transplant 2000;14:70–74.

7 Bromley PN, Cottam SJ, Hilmi I, Tan KC, Heaton N, Ginsburg R, Potter DR: Effects of intraoperative N-acetylcysteine in orthotopic liver transplantation. Br J Anaesth 1995;75:352–354.

8 Thies JC, Teklote J, Clauer U, Tox U, Klar E, Hofmann WJ, Herfarth C, Otto G: The efficacy of N-acetylcysteine as a hepatoprotective agent in liver transplantation. Transpl Int 1998;11(suppl 1):S390–392.

9 Steib A, Freys G, Collin F, Launoy A, Mark G, Boudjema K: Does N-acetylcysteine improve hemodynamics and graft function in liver transplantation? Liver Transpl Surg 1998;4:152–157.

10 Bucuvalas JC, Ryckman FC, Krug S, Alonso MH, Balistreri WF, Kotagal U: Effect of treatment with prostaglandin E1 and N-acetylcysteine on pediatric liver transplant recipients: A single-center study. Pediatr Transplant 2001;5:274–278.

11 Kiemer AK, Baron A, Gerbes AL, Bilzer M, Vollmar AM: The atrial natriuretic peptide as a regulator of Kupffer cell functions. Shock 2002 (in press).

12 Schauer RJ, Bilzer M, Kalmuk S, Gerbes AL, Schildberg FW, Messmer K: Microcirculatory failure after rat liver transplantation is related to Kupffer cell-derived oxidant stress but not involved in early graft dysfunction. Transplantation 2001;72:1692–1699.

13 Bilzer M, Paumgartner G, Gerbes AL: Glutathione protects the rat liver against reperfusion injury after hypothermic preservation. Gastroenterology 1999;117:200–210.

14 Bilzer M, Baron A, Schauer R, Steib C, Ebensberger S, Gerbes AL: Glutathione treatment protects the rat liver against injury after warm ischemia and Kupffer cell activation. Digestion 2002 (in press).

15 Yin DP, Sankary HN, Chong AS, Ma LL, Shen J, Foster P, Williams JW: Protective effect of ischemic preconditioning on liver preservation-reperfusion injury in rats. Transplantation 1998;66: 152–157.

16 Bilzer M, Schauer RJ, Kiemer AK, Baron A, Vollmar AM, Messmer K, Gerbes AL: Potential of preconditioning; in Gerbes AL, et al (eds): Hepatology 2000, Falk Symposium Nr. 117. Lancaster, Kluwer Academic Publishers, 2000, pp 270–278.

17 Gerbes AL, Vollmar AM, Kiemer AK, Bilzer M: The guanylate-cyclase coupled natriuretic peptide (CG-A) receptor – a new target for prevention of cold ischemia-reperfusion damage of the rat liver. Hepatology 1998;28:1309–1317.

18 Kiemer AK, Gerbes AL, Bilzer M, Vollmar AM: The atrial natriuretic peptide and cGMP – novel activators of the heat shock response in rat livers. Hepatology 2002;35:88–94.

19 Bilzer M, Jaeschke H, Vollmar AM, Paumgartner G, Gerbes AL: Prevention of Kupffer cell-induced oxidant injury in rat liver by atrial natriuretic peptide (ANP). Am J Physiol 1999;276: G1137–G1144.

Chirurgische Gastroenterologie Interdisziplinär

Hinweise für Autoren

Chir Gastroenterol 2002;18

Die Zeitschrift CHIRURGISCHE GASTROENTEROLOGIE ist ein Forum für die interdisziplinäre Diskussion aller wichtigen und aktuellen Themen der Viszeralchirurgie, Gastroenterologie und Hepatologie. Alle Beiträge unterliegen einem unabhängigen Begutachtungsverfahren.

1. Allgemeines, Verlagsrecht

Bitte senden Sie Ihr Manuskript in **dreifacher** Ausfertigung (ein Exemplar komplett mit den Originalen der Abbildungen und Tabellen, 2 mit Kopien) an Herrn Prof. Dr. R. Bittner, Marienhospital, Böheimstr. 37, D-70199 Stuttgart, Tel. +49 7 11 64 89 22-01, Fax -13. Eine Kopie des Manuskripts soll grundsätzlich beim Autor verbleiben.

Alle Autoren müssen in einem **Begleitschreiben** durch Unterschrift bestätigen, dass die eingereichte Arbeit bislang weder ganz noch teilweise (Ausnahme: Kongreßberichte) veröffentlicht wurde noch anderweitig zur Veröffentlichung eingereicht ist und dass alle Autoren das Manuskript gelesen haben und mit der Veröffentlichung in der vorliegenden Form einverstanden sind. Es ist Sache des Autors, die Nachdruckerlaubnis für Abbildungen, Tabellen usw. aus anderen Publikationen zu beschaffen. Über die Annahme wissenschaftlicher Beiträge wird aufgrund mehrerer Gutachten entschieden (peer review). Mit der Annahme des Manuskripts gehen alle Rechte auf den Verlag über. Ohne schriftliche Genehmigung des Verlags dürfen diese Publikationen oder Teile daraus nicht in andere Sprachen übersetzt oder in irgendeiner Form mit mechanischen oder elektronischen Mitteln (einschließlich Fotokopie, Tonaufnahme und Mikrofilm) reproduziert oder auf einem Datenträger oder Computersystem gespeichert werden.

Ethische und rechtliche Voraussetzungen: Manuskripte, bei denen Untersuchungen an Probanden oder Patienten durchgeführt wurden, müssen die Erklärung enthalten, dass das Versuchsprotokoll von einer Ethikkommission genehmigt wurde und den ethischen Standards der Deklaration von Helsinki in ihrer erweiterten Form von 1975 und ihren Zusätzen von 1983, 1989 und 1996 [JAMA 1997;277:925–926] entspricht. Zugleich muss im Manuskripttext auf die Einwilligung der Versuchsperson nach Aufklärung hingewiesen werden. Angaben, die auf die Identität der Person schließen lassen, sind unzulässig. Tierversuche bedürfen gleichfalls der Genehmigung und müssen den Forderungen des Tierschutzgesetzes in seiner jeweils gültigen Fassung entsprechen. Auf diese Genehmigung ist im Manuskript hinzuweisen. Arbeiten, die nicht aus Deutschland stammen, müssen einen vergleichbaren Hinweis tragen.

Rubriken: Beiträge erscheinen als Beiträge zum Hauptthema, Interdiziplinäres Gespräch, Originalarbeiten, Übersichtsarbeiten und als Arbeiten zur Prä- und Postoperativen Therapie sowie Minimal invasiven Chirurgie.

2. Manuskripte

Die Manuskripte sollen in 1½zeiligem Abstand mit beidseitig 3 cm Rand ausgedruckt werden. Originalarbeiten sollten 5 Druckseiten (zirka 15 Manuskriptseiten einschl. Literatur und Tabellen) nicht überschreiten. Für Umfangsüberschreitungen wird dem Autor ein Mehrkostenanteil in Rechnung gestellt (s. u.). Kontrollieren Sie das Manuskript sorgfältig auf einheitliche Bezeichnung und korrekte Schreibweise. Typographische Gestaltung und redaktionelle Bearbeitung werden vom Verlag durchgeführt. Generelle Hinweise zur Abfassung von Manuskripten können den «Uniform Requirements for Manuscripts Submitted to Biomedical Journals» des «International Committee of Medical Journal Editors», veröffentlicht in Ann Intern Med 1997;126:36–47. bzw. http://jama.asma_assn.org/info/auinst_reg.html, entnommen werden.

Manuskripte auf Diskette: Dem zur Veröffentlichung angenommenen Manuskript **muss** eine Diskette beigelegt werden, deren Inhalt exakt mit dem Ausdruck übereinstimmen muß. Bitte beachten Sie auch die «Hinweise für Abgabe von Manuskripten auf Diskette».

Die Seiten des Manuskripts müssen, beginnend mit der Titelseite, durchlaufend nummeriert sein. Die Arbeit soll gegliedert sein in **Schlüsselwörter** und **Zusammenfassung, Key Words** und **Summary**, **Einleitung, Material und Methoden** (oder **Patienten und Methoden**), **Ergebnisse, Diskussion,** gegebenenfalls **Dank, Literatur, Tabellen, Abbildungslegenden** und **Abbildungen**.

Die **Titelseite** muss enthalten: **Titel und Kurztitel** der Arbeit in Deutsch und Englisch, die vollständigen Autorennamen mit der jeweiligen Institutsangabe o.ä. in der Landessprache der Autoren, die vollständige Postadresse des Korrespondenzautors mit Telefon- und Faxnummer sowie der E-mail-Adresse.

Alle Arbeiten müssen eine englische und deutsche **Zusammenfassung** (max. 250 Wörter) sowie 3–5 **Schlüsselwörter** (Englisch und Deutsch) enthalten, die möglichst der «Medical Subjects Heading List» des Index Medicus entnommen sein sollen (die Liste ist unter www.nlm.nih.gov erhältlich). Die Zusammenfassung darf keine Literaturzitate, Tabellen, Abbildungen, Abbildungs- und Tabellenhinweise enthalten. Unvermeidliche Hinweise auf Literaturzitate müssen vollständig sein.

Fußnoten sollten nur in Tabellen verwendet werden. Abkürzungen bitte möglichst sparsam verwenden. Bei speziellen **Abkürzungen** jeweils beim ersten Auftreten das Wort ausschreiben und die später verwendete Abkürzung in Klammern folgen lassen: z. B. Adenosin-Monophosphat (AMP). Geschützte **Produkt- bzw. Markennamen** müssen beim ersten Auftreten im Text mit einem hochgestellten ® bzw. ™ bezeichnet werden. Die Verantwortung für die korrekte Befolgung dieser Vorschrift liegt ausschließlich beim Autor. **Danksagungen** sollten unmittelbar dem Text folgen und dem Literaturverzeichnis vorangestellt sein.

Das **Literaturverzeichnis** soll nur die im Text zitierten Publikationen enthalten. Die Literatur ist entsprechend der Reihenfolge des Auftretens im Text zu nummerieren. Die Referenzen werden als Zahlen in eckigen Klammern in den Text eingefügt. Bitte alle Autoren einer Arbeit angeben, die Abkürzung «et al.» ist zu vermeiden. Es sollten nur Arbeiten zitiert werden, die entweder publiziert oder zur Publikation angenommen wurden. Der Hinweis «in Vorbereitung» oder «persönliche Mitteilung» ist zu vermeiden. Die Abkürzung der Zeitschriftentitel erfolgt nach dem Index-Medicus-System (http://www.nlm.nih.gov).

Zur Abfassung von Literaturzitaten gelten folgende Beispiele:

(a) Zeitschriftenbeiträge: Lelie PN, Cuypers HTM, van Drimmelen AAJ, Quint WGV: Quality assessment of hepatitis C virus nucleic acid amplification methods. An international proficiency study. Infusionsther Transfusionsmed 1998;25:102-110.

(b) Bücher mit Herausgeber: Hardy WD Jr, Essex M: FeLV-induced feline acquired immune deficiency syndrome: A model for human AIDS; in Klein E (ed): Acquired Immunodeficiency Syndrome. Prog Allergy. Basel, Karger, 1986, vol 37, pp 353-376.

(c) Monographien: Schaefer UW, Beelen DW: Bone Marrow Transplantation, ed 2, revised. Basel, Karger, 1996.

In **Abbildungen** und **Tabellen** genannte Informationen bedürfen keiner Wiederholung im Text. Hinweise auf Abbildungen und Tabellen erfolgen im Text mit (Abb. 1) bzw. (Tab. 1). Abbildungslegenden sind auf einer gesonderten Seite zusammenzustellen. Die Legenden der Tabellen und Abbildungen sind kurz und präzise abzufassen. **Farbabbildungen** sind möglich, erfordern jedoch einen Zuschuß des Autors zu den Druckkosten (s. u.). **Abbildungsvorlagen** sind 3fach einzureichen (Original und 2 Kopien). Auf der Rückseite der Vorlage (nicht aufkleben oder anheften) bitte den Namen des Autors, ein Titelstichwort, die Angabe, wo «oben» ist, sowie die Bildnummer angeben. Die Qualität der gedruckten Abbildungen hängt von der Qualität der Vorlagen ab.

Druckfahnen: Das lektorierte Manuskript und die Druckfahnen werden dem Korrespondenzautor zusammen mit einem Formular zur Sonderdruckbestellung zugeschickt. Die Fahnen sind mit dem Manuskript zu vergleichen und notwendige Korrekturen auf der Fahne einzutragen. Die Korrespondenz betreffend angenommene Arbeiten und Druckfahnen bitte direkt mit der S. Karger GmbH, Verlagsbüro Leipzig, Dr. Hannelore Tenckhoff, Querstr. 18, D-04103 Leipzig führen.

3. Kosten und Sonderdrucke

a) Übersteigen die Kosten der Autorkorrektur 10% der Satzkosten, werden die Zusatzkosten dem Autor in Rechnung gestellt.
b) Sollte die Arbeit den vorgegebenen Umfang überschreiten und vom Autor nicht gekürzt werden, wird der Mehrumfang mit Euro 335,– plus MWSt. pro Druckseite berechnet.
c) Für Farbabbildungen wird dem Autor ein Reproduktions- und Druckkostenanteil von Euro 235,– plus MWSt. pro Abbildung in Rechnung gestellt.

Der Korrespondenzautor erhält 25 kostenlose Sonderdrucke seiner Arbeit (gilt nicht für Supplemente).

Die vollständigen Hinweise erscheinen im ersten Heft eines Jahrgangs.

Hinweise für Manuskripte auf Diskette

Bitte reichen Sie zusammen mit dem Manuskript eine Diskette ein. Prüfen Sie die Diskette mit einem Virensuchprogramm. Der Inhalt der Diskette **muss exakt** mit dem beigelegten Ausdruck übereinstimmen. Bitte vermeiden Sie das Komprimieren der Dateien mit einem Packprogramm. Auf dem Etikett der Diskette müssen folgende Angaben vermerkt sein: Titel der Arbeit, Name des Erstautors, sowie verwendetes Betriebssystem und Software (Versionsnummer). Sowohl Disketten im Macintosh-Format als auch MS-DOS-formatierte Disketten werden akzeptiert. Speichern Sie den Text in dem vom Textverarbeitungsprogramm angebotenen Standardformat ab. Das bevorzugte Textverarbeitungsprogramm ist MS-Word. Dateien anderer verbreiteter Textverarbeitungsprogramme sowie ASCII-Formate können ebenfalls bearbeitet werden. Die Datei sollte keine Seitenlayout-Anweisungen, wie Hinweise zur Plazierung von Grafiken, enthalten. Bitte den Text linksbündig schreiben und keine Silbentrennungen durchführen. Erfassen Sie Ihren Text endlos, d. h. benutzen Sie harte Zeilenschaltungen (Return-Taste) nur am Ende eines Absatzes oder für Titel, Untertitel usw. Bitte verwenden Sie **nur ein Format** (Normal) für die Erstellung des Textes. Dateien, die aufwendig formatiert sind, können nur unter Schwierigkeiten in das Satzprogramm übernommen werden. Zur Gliederung des Textes können Tabulatoren verwendet werden, Kopf- und Fußzeilen bitte vermeiden. Prüfen Sie, ob die folgenden Zeichen im Manuskript korrekt wiedergegeben sind: 1 (Eins) und l (Buchstabe), 0 (null) und O (Buchstabe), X (Buchstabe) und × (Malkreuz). Tabellen und Abbildungen sollen nicht in den Text integriert werden, bitte speichern Sie diese als separate Dateien (siehe auch «Abbildungen»). Bitte fügen Sie keinen Leerschlag vor dem Punkt ein. Es wird die Verwendung der Schriften Times und Symbol empfohlen.

Abbildungen

Illustrationen jeder Art sollten als separate Datei gespeichert werden. Die meisten der für die Erstellung der Abbildungen verwendeten Programme erlauben die Speicherung in verschiedenen Dateiformaten. TIFF, PostScript oder EPS werden bevorzugt. Die Abbildung sollte anhand des Dateinamens zugeordnet werden können. Zusätzlich **müssen** alle Abbildungen unbedingt als reprofähige Vorlagen mitgeliefert werden.

Literatur

Bitte beachten Sie für die Abfassung der Literatur die «Hinweise für Autoren». Verwenden Sie kein Komma nach dem Nachnamen und keine Punkte nach den Initialen. Nach Semikolon und Doppelpunkt darf kein Leerschlag eingefügt werden, *falsch:* Infusionsther Transfusionsmed 1998; 25: 160 - 3., *richtig:* Infusionsther Transfusionsmed 1998;25:160–163.

KARGER

Fax +49 761 452 07 14
E-mail Information@Karger.de
www.karger.com

Hinweise für Autoren verfügbar unter:
www.karger.com/journals/cga/cga_gl.htm

Interdisziplinär – Aktuell – Informativ

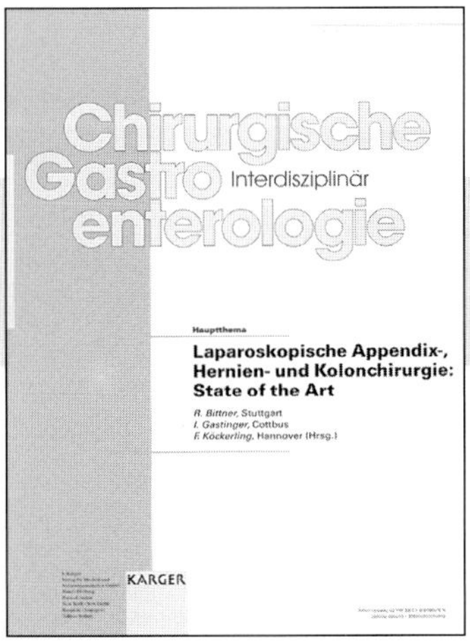

Chirurgische Gastroenterologie Interdisziplinär

Hauptschriftleitung
R. Bittner, *Stuttgart*

Schriftleitung
Viszeralchirurgie
E. Klar, *Heidelberg*

Schriftleitung
Gastroenterologie
J. Mössner, *Leipzig*

Assistenz Schriftleitung
C.-G. Schmedt, *Stuttgart*

Fachschriftleitung
H. Bosseckert, *Jena*
C.E. Broelsch, *Essen*
H.P. Bruch, *Lübeck*
M.W. Büchler, *Bern*
I. Gastinger, *Cottbus*
K. Glaser, *Wien*
J. Hauss, *Leipzig*
J.R. Izbicki, *Hamburg*
H. Lippert, *Magdeburg*
K.-J. Paquet, *Hannover*
H. Säuberli, *Baden*
R. Schiessel, *Wien*
B. Ulrich, *Düsseldorf*
W.G. Zoller, *Stuttgart*

Einsenden von Arbeiten

Originalarbeiten in deutscher und englischer Sprache werden veröffentlicht.

Manuskripte sind zu senden an:

Prof. Dr. R. Bittner
Marienhospital
Böheimstr. 37
D–70199 Stuttgart
(Deutschland)

Lesen Sie's Online:
www.karger.com/journals/cga

Ihr Direktzugang zu Volltext-artikeln, Online-Reprints, Inhalts-verzeichnissen – mit freiem Zugriff auf Abstracts, Probenummern und auf E-mail ToC-Alert service.

Diese Zeitschrift ist die einzige Publikation, die sich mit interdisziplinärer Gastroenterologie in Klinik, Praxis und Forschung befasst. In eingeladenen Beiträgen wird unter der redaktionellen Verantwortung eines namhaften Klinikers zu einem aktuellen Thema Stellung genommen. Gastroenterologen, Internisten, Radiologen, Allgemein-, Gefäss- und Abdominalchirurgen finden im Teil «Interdisziplinäre Gespräche» Antwort auf praxisbezogene Fragen. In weiteren Rubriken werden Originalarbeiten publiziert sowie Trends der prä- und postoperativen Therapie und minimalinvasiven Chirurgie vorgestellt. Buchbesprechungen und Industrieneuheiten ergänzen die jeweilige Ausgabe. Zusätzlich erscheinen Supplemente zu aktuellen Problemen. Somit werden die wesentlichen Erkenntnisse der gesamten chirurgischen Gastroenterologie der letzten 10 Jahre behandelt; die Zeitschrift hat damit auch die Funktion eines hochaktuellen Lehrbuchs.

Eine Auswahl repräsentativer Beiträge

Die endoskopische Leistenhernienreparation im Vergleich zu offenen Operationsverfahren: Was ist Evidence-basiert? Eine systematische Literaturübersicht randomisierter Studien: ***Schmedt, C.-G.; Leibl, B.J.; Bittner, R.*** *(Stuttgart)*

Laparoskopische versus offene Appendektomie: Was ist gesichert?: ***Uhl, W.; Strobel, O.; Büchler, M.W.*** *(Bern)*

Ergebnisse der laparoskopischen kolorektalen Chirurgie: ***Scheuerlein, H.; Scheidbach, H.; Schneider, C.; Diddens, H.; Köckerling, F.*** *(Hannover)*

Welcher endoskopisch abgetragene Kolonpolyp bedarf einer zusätzlichen onkochirurgischen Kolonresektion?: ***Netzer, P.; Knoblauch, C.; Göke, B.*** *(Bern)*

Neue Techniken der Kontinenzerhaltung beim tiefsitzenden Rektumkarzinom ***Kasperk, R.; Willis, S.; Schumpelick, V.*** *(Aachen)*

Adjuvante Chemotherapie des Kolonkarzinoms – ein Update: ***Porschen, R.*** *(Bremen);* ***Nehls, O.*** *(Tübingen)*

Strategie der kombinierten minimalenteralen und parenteralen Ernährung des kritisch Kranken: ***Suchner, U.; Felbinger, T.W.; Sachs, M.; Goetz, A.E.; Peter, K.*** *(München)*

Bedeutung des Rekonstruktionsverfahrens für die Ernährung und Lebensqualität nach Gastrektomie: ***Lehnert, T.; Maksan, S.M.; Kienle, P.; Buhl, K.; Herfarth, C.*** *(Heidelberg)*

Chirurgische Gastroenterologie
2002: Band 18 mit 4 Heften
Sprachen: Deutsch, Englisch
ISSN 0177–9990
Aufgeführt in bibliographischen Diensten und in *Reference Update, EMBASE/Excerpta Medica.*

Preise für Studenten und Ärzte in Weiterbildung

Abonnement	+ Versandkosten	
CHF 101.–	+ CHF 19.20	Europa
CHF 101.–	+ CHF 28.50	Übersee
EUR 72.–	+ EUR 11.–	
USD 77.50	+ USD 19.20	

+ Online-Abonnement pro Band:
CHF 39.– / EUR 28.– / USD 30.00

Abonnementspreise

Abonnement	+ Versandkosten	
CHF 202.–	+ CHF 24.–	Europa
CHF 202.–	+ CHF 35.60	Übersee
EUR 144.–	+ EUR 11.–	
USD 155.00	+ USD 24.00	

+ Online-Abonnement pro Band:
CHF 58.– / EUR 42.– / USD 45.00

Preisänderungen vorbehalten
EUR-Preis nur für Deutschland,
USD-Preis nur für USA

KARGER

Verlangen Sie ein kostenloses Probeheft!

KF 02015